FINDING YOUR FLOW IN THE FIRST WEEKS OF BREASTFEEDING

MILK'D

NAIOMI S. CATRON

Milk'D: Finding Your Flow in the First Weeks of Breastfeeding

For permissions or bulk orders, contact: www.milkdbook.com

Disclaimer

If you believe you are experiencing a medical emergency, please call 911 immediately.

The information contained within this book is intended for educational and informational purposes only and should not be mistaken for medical advice. The content is not a substitute for professional medical guidance, diagnosis, or treatment. Readers are strongly encouraged to consult with a licensed medical doctor or qualified healthcare professional regarding any medical concerns or questions related to their health or the health of their baby.

The author and publisher assume no liability for any medical issues, complications, or outcomes that may arise as a result of applying the information presented in this book.

Please note that the content of this book is based on resources and research available as of 2024. Medical research and recommendations are constantly evolving, and some of the information in this book may become outdated as new discoveries emerge. Always consult up-to-date, evidence-based sources and seek advice from medical professionals to ensure the best care for you and your baby.

ISBN: 979-8-9925464-0-8
First edition: 2025
Author: Naiomi S. Catron
Cover design by: Anze Ban V
Edited by: Write & Main
Published by: Oxytocin Publishing
Printed in the United States of America

To my pregnant past self—

Full of dreams, strength, and anticipation, yet completely unaware of how motherhood would forever reshape her identity.

And to every pregnant woman standing on the edge of transformation—

Glowing with excitement and love, not yet knowing how quickly that joy can become tangled with self-doubt and feelings of not being enough—This book is for you.

May you find grace in your journey, comfort in your chaos, and the reminder that you were never meant to do this alone.

TABLE OF CONTENTS

PART III: WHAT I WISH I'D KNOWN IN THE FIRST WEEKS

A MESSAGE TO YOU

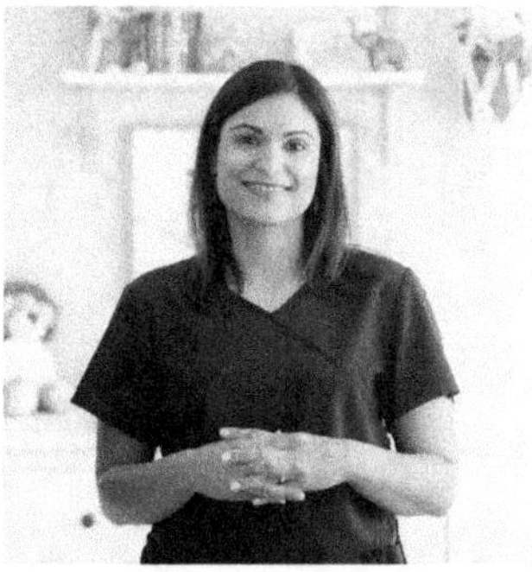

If you're holding this book, you're either preparing for your first breastfeeding experience or hoping *this* time will be different. Whether you're feeling a mix of excitement and uncertainty or carrying the weight of a previous struggle, you're not alone in this amazing, messy, beautiful journey.

As the founder of Milk Diva Lactation Services and an International Board-Certified Lactation Consultant (IBCLC), I've guided thousands of families through their breastfeeding journeys. And I've learned that having the right knowledge in those first two weeks can be the difference between stressing over every ounce and confidently feeding your baby.

My journey—from struggling first-time mom to award-winning labor and delivery nurse to leading one of the most trusted lactation practices in Austin, Texas—has taught me the things I wish every mother knew from the start. What makes the biggest difference isn't the basic how-tos of breastfeeding—it's the insider knowledge that usually only comes with experience. That's why this book focuses on those crucial first fourteen days, sharing the exact insights you need, right when you need them most, with a touch of humor along the way.

Drawing from both my personal experience and thousands of clinical hours supporting new mothers, I've distilled exactly what you need to know to start your breastfeeding journey with confidence. Every recommendation in this book comes from real conversations, real challenges, and real solutions—tested and refined through years of practice with thousands of mothers and babies. Let's dive in together, and remember: You've got this, and I've got you.

Warmly,
Naiomi S. Catron, RN, IBCLC
Founder, Milk Diva

INTRODUCTION

When my first baby was born, the iPhone hadn't been invented yet—no Instagram, no Facebook. I don't even know if Google was a popular place to do research. My husband and I were completely on our own, trying to figure everything out in California while my entire family was back in New York. Not only was I away from my family, but I was navigating entirely new territory—I was the first one in my family to breastfeed.

For the women in my family, breastfeeding hadn't been a realistic option. It was a privilege they couldn't access. They had to return to work immediately, couldn't afford pumps or help, and were led to believe formula was best. But I had an opportunity they never had, and I was determined to breastfeed. What I didn't realize was how hard it would be to figure out on my own.

With no family experience to draw from and no online resources to turn to, I struggled to understand what was "normal" and what wasn't. (If only I'd had a podcast back then—though I probably would've been too tired to find the play button!) My baby was skinny and jaundiced. He seemed hungry every sixty minutes, all day and all night long. He was yellow, and because of our skin tone, I didn't realize there was a problem until his eyes also turned yellow. Meanwhile, I watched my two good friends breastfeed their babies with no hiccups while I couldn't, for the life of me, figure out why my experience was so different.

Looking back now, I wish someone had told me some crucial things from the start. For instance, it would've been helpful to know it can take time for a baby to properly latch and transfer milk, especially when factors like medication or health conditions are involved. Like many new mothers, I'd assumed babies just naturally latch and feed on their own. (That's what usually happens in the movies.)

I also wish I'd known how different breastfeeding is for a late preterm baby and how that can cause problems with your milk supply. That was my experience, and it is definitely a struggle when you want to immediately breastfeed your newborn but the milk volume isn't there yet. And I really wish someone had talked to me about bottles differently. Instead of just being warned about using a bottle and causing 'nipple confusion,' I needed to know that babies are actually pretty smart about feeding. If bottles become part of your journey, there are ways to use them that can actually complement breastfeeding rather than hurt it.

Since I didn't have any of this information, my struggle with low milk supply led me down a tough path. I ended up triple feeding for six months—breastfeeding, then bottle feeding, then pumping for every single feed. Picture trying to juggle three different feeding methods while operating on two hours of sleep: it's like trying to perform a circus act in slow motion, except your audience is a tiny human who's already gearing up for the next show. I think it goes without saying, but it's something I would *never* recommend to anyone today. It stole the joy of having a baby. I missed those important periods because I was so focused on the volume of milk I was making. That's why I have a sign in my office that says:

"Your worth is not measured in ounces."

This experience changed everything for me. It's one of the reasons I became a lactation consultant, and it's why I'm writing this book. Those first weeks of breastfeeding might feel like a sprint, but finding your flow is more like settling into a marathon pace. It's moving past those early moments of "I wish someone had told me" to a place where you and your baby are in sync. Where feeding doesn't steal your joy. Where you're not constantly comparing your journey to others or wrestling with self-doubt. The first two weeks are pivotal to help set the stage for this transition to happen.

The Mom Journey: What I Wish Someone Would Have Told Me

I want to make one thing clear: this book isn't about the basics of breastfeeding, decoding your newborn's behaviors, or mastering nursing positions. It's a collection of aha moments that countless mothers have shared over the years, moments when they've exclaimed, "I wish I'd known this before!" I'll be your trusted guide, helping you navigate the unexpected twists and turns of your baby's first few weeks, all while keeping your long-term feeding goals firmly intact.

Throughout this book, you'll find **Mom-to-Mom Insights**—special moments where I share real-life experiences and reflections from mothers who have navigated these same waters.

You'll also find **Rules of Thumb**—quick, practical tips that you can rely on during those sleep-deprived early days. Like a friend's advice scribbled on a sticky note, these Rules of Thumb are bite-sized bits of wisdom you can quickly reference when you need them most.

Finally, sprinkled throughout these pages, you'll discover **Insider Secrets**—professional insights I've gathered from working with thousands of breastfeeding mothers that rarely appear in standard resources. These are the subtle, game-changing observations that experienced lactation consultants notice but seldom have the opportunity to widely share.

Answering Your Most Pressing Questions

With these resources at your fingertips, we can address the questions that keep new mothers up at night (in addition to their hungry babies). Like me, you might be wondering if your experience is normal. Are you the only one struggling with a painful latch? Is it okay that your baby wants to feed so often? Should you be worried about your milk supply? In the chapters ahead, we'll explore these questions together, sharing the kind of honest, practical advice I wish I'd had in those early days. No more guessing, no more second-guessing—just real talk about what to expect and when to get help.

Speaking of wishes, here's another lesson I learned the hard way: breastfeeding isn't about perfection—it's about progress. Those first weeks might feel like you're racing against time, trying to get everything right. But just like my journey from struggling mom to lactation consultant, your path will have its own unique challenges and victories. And that's okay.

I see it in my practice every day. Moms compare their feeding journey to what they see on social media or hear from other mothers. But here's the truth: every baby is different, every mother is different, and every feeding journey is different. The sooner we embrace this, the sooner we can focus on what really matters: finding what works for you and your baby. Because confidence in feeding doesn't come from matching someone else's experience; it comes from discovering your own path forward.

You're more than capable of navigating this journey and embracing the narrative of your unique story. And you don't have to figure it all out alone. Through my clinical practice and hosting The Boob Business Podcast, I've heard thousands of mothers share their "I wish I had known" moments. Each story has reinforced what I learned the hard way: preparation is everything. So, let's venture forward together and get you ready for your baby's first few weeks of life!

Rule of Thumb: Speaking of preparation, you'll want to schedule a prenatal lactation consultation or class between weeks 28–34 of pregnancy. Don't wait until after your baby arrives. This single step can prevent weeks of stress and struggle.

Mom-to-Mom Insight: "I wish I had seen a lactation consultant [LC] outside of the hospital sooner. I triple fed for three months, and while it was worth it, it was exhausting, and I believe seeing an LC sooner would have cut that time down and made my breastfeeding journey easier." —L.G.

PART I:

WHAT I WISH I'D KNOWN BEFORE BIRTH

CHAPTER 1:

BOSS-LEVEL PREP FOR BREASTFEEDING SUCCESS

I wish I'd known...

Nature gave us the equipment for breastfeeding. It just didn't give us the manual. And with thousands of hours of feeding ahead, you deserve better prep than just "You'll figure it out, mama."

Embarking on a breastfeeding journey is like setting off for a grand hike in a national park—except your hiking partner is a newborn who hasn't read the trail guide. While you've spent months preparing for the big event—gathering supplies, reading books, watching videos—nothing quite prepares you for that moment when you're actually on the trail with your tiny adventurer.

Your baby, unlike a typical hiking buddy, can't tell you, "Hey, this path isn't working" or "I need a snack break." Instead, they communicate through a series of cues that can feel about as clear as trying to read a trail map in the dark. And what about the lactation support you were told would be available after birth? Well, the reality is more like showing up to find just two park rangers trying to help several dozen hikers at once. Those hospital lactation consultants are amazing professionals, but they're often stretched thinner than a worn-out backpack strap—just two consultants caring for forty to sixty patients in some hospitals. That's barely enough time for them to point you in the right direction, let alone teach you all the skills you'll need for the journey ahead.

So there you are, smartphone in hand, frantically googling "how to tell my baby got enough milk" while trying to decode your little one's hunger signs. (Sound familiar? I've been there, desperately searching "how often to feed a newborn" at 3 A.M.) Your perfectly planned hike suddenly feels more like an unexpected obstacle course, complete with challenges you never saw coming—like a super-sleepy baby who treats feeding time like nap time, or nipples that feel like they've gone through their own endurance test.

Well, say hello to your expert "hiking guide"!

As your trusted hiking guide, I'm honored to lead you through the winding trails of your breastfeeding journey. Think of me as your personal guide who's not only walked these trails before but has helped thousands of other parents navigate them too. Think of me as the friend who knows all the shortcuts, has packed extra trail mix, and won't judge you for asking the same question five times. (Because let's be honest, sleep deprivation makes us all a little forgetful!)

Birth Prep vs. Breastfeeding Prep

When I was pregnant with my first, I spent weeks crafting the nursery and picking the perfect stroller. But you know what never made it onto my planning checklist? A breastfeeding plan. Like most new moms, I had no idea what I was in for and I assumed breastfeeding would come naturally.

A typical newborn feeds approximately eight to twelve times a day, sometimes even more frequently. That translates to numerous precious moments spent nourishing and bonding with your baby. Over the course of a week, it amounts to fifty-six to eighty-four feeding sessions. Extend it to a month, and you're looking at roughly 240 to 360 breastfeeding sessions. Over a year, well, you're talking about thousands of feedings and tens of thousands of hours!

Here's what gets me: we spend months preparing for childbirth—an event that lasts hours or maybe a couple of days—but barely think about breastfeeding, which we'll be doing thousands of times. Don't misunderstand; giving birth is undoubtedly a monumental event. Labor and delivery can last anywhere from a few hours to a day or two, with the actual birthing process often measured in minutes. But when you compare all the time we spend preparing for birth to how little we prepare for breastfeeding, something doesn't add up. We invest months in prenatal classes, birthing workshops, and meticulously planned delivery experiences. Yet how much of that preparation focuses on breastfeeding—something we'll be doing multiple times every day for months or even years? It's like spending hours researching how to find the trailhead parking lot without preparing for the hike ahead.

This isn't me being dramatic about preparation. Multiple studies have shed light on an intriguing discovery: prenatal breastfeeding education significantly elevates the rate of exclusive breastfeeding at the six-month mark, perfectly aligning with global health guidelines. But this isn't just a matter of statistics. It's about you feeling confident and prepared when you're up in the middle of the night with your newborn. It's about having tools ready to overcome challenges like latch issues or engorgement *before* they happen. Think of this book as your investment in smoother nights, easier days, and a whole lot more confidence in your breastfeeding journey.

Mom-to-Mom Insight: "The beginning is truly the hardest. You are both learning how to do this thing, and it isn't instinctual or necessarily "natural" at first. Give yourself grace; reach out for support. If you can make it two days, you can make it two weeks. If you can make it two weeks, you can make it two months. And then before you know it, time will have passed in the blink of an eye and it will be time to end your journey. Whether you've loved the process or not, it's part of your story. Part of your legacy to your baby. And know that you don't have to love every second of nursing (and/or pumping). Let it be enough. You are enough, exactly as you are. Be so proud of every second, every milliliter you offer your baby. You got this, mama! We are all cheering you on." —former patient Mary Beth O'Connell

The Impact of Breastfeeding: Unveiling the Evidence

Now, let's chat about something truly extraordinary: the astonishing benefits of breastfeeding. It's not merely about choosing how to feed your baby. It's about embracing an experience that's scientifically proven to be profoundly beneficial for both you and your little one. Before we dive into the advantages of breastfeeding, let's address the common misconception that breastfeeding will come easily because it's natural. It stems from the notion that breastfeeding should unfold effortlessly, like a spontaneous act of maternal magic. But the truth is, breastfeeding is more than instinct—it's a skill, an art form, and, occasionally, a bit of science. It requires knowledge, practice, and skilled support.

The Impact for Your Little One

- **Immune Boost: A Shield Against Infections**
  Think of your breast milk as your baby's first superpower, keeping them healthy and strong. Breast milk is packed with antibodies, living cells, and enzymes that provide unmatched protection.[1] It's like giving them a powerful shield against infections and illnesses right from day one. Babies fed breast milk tend to experience significantly fewer infections during infancy.

1 "Making the Decision to Breastfeed." Making the Decision to Breastfeed | Office on Women's Health, www.womenshealth.gov/breastfeeding/making-decision-breastfeed. Accessed 4 Sept. 2024.

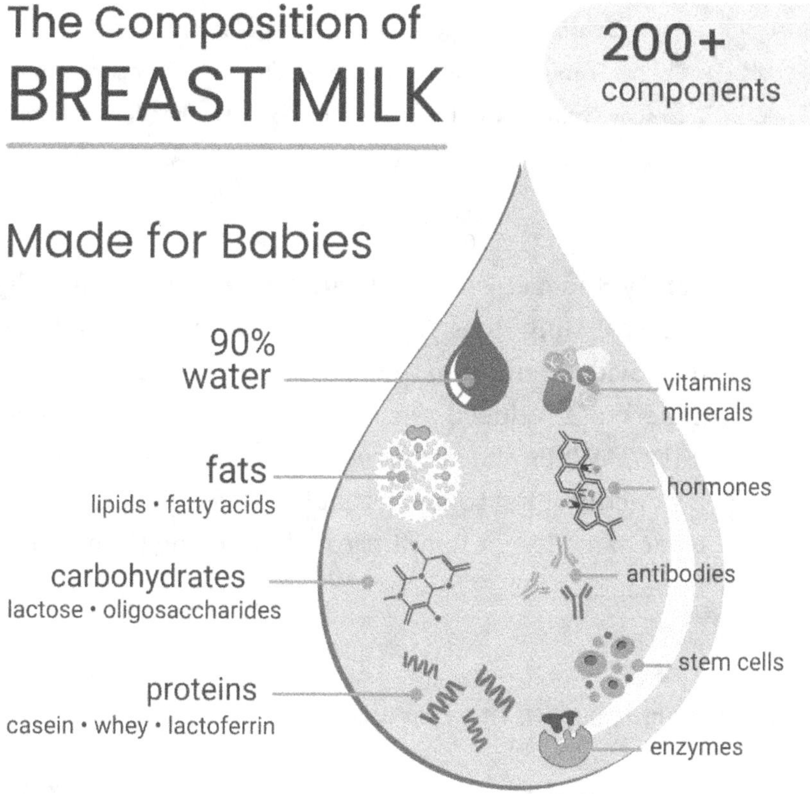

- **Growth Serum: Tailored Nutrition for Your Baby**
  Breast milk isn't just any milk; it's a tailor-made potion of nutrients designed exclusively for your baby. It's like a personalized growth elixir that fosters sturdy brain development. As your baby grows, breast milk adapts its composition to match their evolving needs. Whether it's proteins, fats, or carbohydrates, every drop contains a piece of the puzzle for your baby's growth, providing them with the best possible start in life.

Rule of Thumb: Trust your body's superpower to customize your milk. You don't need diet changes or supplements to make your milk "better." Your body is already adapting its composition to match exactly what your baby needs right now, whether they're fighting a cold or hitting a growth spurt.

- **Safety Snooze: Peace of Mind for You and Your Baby**
  Breastfeeding doesn't just bring about physical benefits—it provides emotional peace too. Breastfeeding has been linked to a reduced risk of sudden infant death syndrome (SIDS).[2] While the exact reasons are still being researched, it's encouraging to know that breastfeeding offers an extra layer of safety for your little one, allowing them to slumber in peace.

The Impact for You, the Heroic Mom

- **Postpartum Resilience: Bouncing Back Faster**
  After the roller coaster of childbirth, your body deserves a superhero's recovery. Breastfeeding is like a reset button, helping your uterus shrink back down to its prepregnancy size more swiftly.[3] It's almost like a postpartum workout for your body. This not only speeds up your recovery but also reduces postpartum bleeding.[4]

---

2 *Breastfeed Your Baby to Reduce the Risk of* SIDS, National Institute of Child Health and Human Development , www.nichd.nih.gov/sites/default/files/2018-11/Breastfeed_Baby_SIDS_final.pdf. Accessed 27 May 2024.

3 World Journal of Research and Review (WJRR), "Effect of Breastfeeding on Uterine Involution and Postpartum Recovery," Volume 9, Issue 2, 2023.

4 "Relief of Pain Caused by Uterine Cramping or Involution After Giving Birth," published October 20, 2020.

- **Calorie Burning: A Weight-Loss Companion**
  Breastfeeding is like having a built-in calorie-burning mechanism. While you're nourishing your baby, you're also expending extra calories—about 300 to 400 per day.[5] This is a dual benefit that makes managing your post-pregnancy weight more achievable. It's a healthy and natural way to get back to feeling like yourself, one step at a time.

- **Cancer Prevention: Reducing Your Health Risks**
  Breastfeeding isn't just about protecting your baby. It also offers you a shield against certain health risks. Research indicates that breastfeeding can reduce your chances of developing breast and ovarian cancer by 24–34%, with the extent of risk reduction depending on factors such as the total duration of breastfeeding.[6][7] It's like an added layer of defense for you, empowering you to lead a healthier life and enjoy motherhood without the shadows of these health concerns.

- **Oxytocin Oasis: Strengthening the Bond**
  Beyond the physical benefits, there's also the emotional benefit of breastfeeding: the release of oxytocin, the bonding hormone. During breastfeeding, oxytocin flows freely, weaving a strong maternal connection with your baby. It's like a love potion that brings you closer to your little one. Breastfeeding creates moments of intimacy and love that strengthen the connection between you and your baby, nurturing them in more ways than one.

---

5 UPMC HealthBeat, "How Much Energy Does Breastfeeding Take?" UPMC, May 22, 2023

6 Australian researchers, "Duration of Breastfeeding and Risk Reduction of Breast Cancer and Ovarian Cancer," International Journal of Cancer Epidemiology, vol. 45, no. 3 (2024): 563–575, accessed April 8, 2025, https://onlinelibrary.wiley.com/doi/10.1155/2024/1987378.

7 Lindsey Wohlford, "Breastfeeding Lowers Your Breast Cancer Risk," MD Anderson Cancer Center, last modified October 9, 2014, accessed April 8, 2025, https://www.mdanderson.org/publications/focused-on-health/breastfeeding-breast-cancer-prevention.h19-1589046.html.

The Money-Saving Angle

But hold onto your capes; there's more. Breastfeeding isn't just a health superhero, it's an economic wizard. Research shows that breastfeeding can curb medical bills due to fewer illnesses, clinic visits, and hospital stays. Plus, providing your breast milk to your baby can trim your budget by eliminating the cost of formula—which could cost more than $150 per month (as of 2025, with costs varying by brand and region).

"Recent research shows that if 90 percent of families breastfed exclusively for 6 months, nearly 1,000 deaths among infants could be prevented. The United States would also save $13 billion per year; medical care costs are lower for fully breastfed infants than never breastfed infants. Breastfed infants typically need fewer sick care visits, prescriptions, and hospitalizations."[8]

When I talk to families about the cost of formula, their eyes often go wide. But what really gets them is adding up all those potential medical visits and prescriptions we can avoid. It's like having both a superhero power and a magic money-saving wand!

Finding Your Flow: The Journey Begins with Knowledge

With these compelling reasons, it's clear that breastfeeding is more than a short-term choice; it's a dynamic health decision that ripples through time and generations. Yet, here's the kicker: studies suggest that many mothers fall short of their breastfeeding

8 "Making the Decision to Breastfeed." *Making the Decision to Breastfeed | Office on Women's Health*, www.womenshealth.gov/breastfeeding/making-decision-breastfeed. Accessed 27 May 2024.

goals, often due to insufficient support and preparation.[9][10][11] If you're reading this book, you're already on your way to overcoming that obstacle! And I'm here to help you write your own superhero success story.

As we prepare for this journey together, remember that while the benefits are clear, the path isn't always easy. That's why I want to share one final thought from a mother who's been there:

> **Mom-to-Mom Insight:** "Though breastfeeding is natural, it is not a skill that you are born with but one that must be acquired through time and patience."
> —former patient Zulmy Galindo

9 PubMed Central, "Reasons for Earlier Than Desired Cessation of Breastfeeding," published February 18, 2013

10 ACOG (American College of Obstetricians and Gynecologists), "Barriers to Breastfeeding: Supporting Initiation and Continuation of Breastfeeding," published February 2021.

11 Sage Journals, "Mothers' Experiences of Breastfeeding Support and Specialists' Views on Breastfeeding Promotion," published June 4, 2024

CHAPTER 2:

YOUR BOOBS, YOUR RULES, YOUR JOURNEY

I wish I'd known...

Successful breastfeeding isn't having everything figured out from day one. You have to take a week-by-week approach, celebrate the small victories, and find your own path. It's all about progress, not perfection.

Let me make something crystal clear before we venture further into this breastfeeding journey: this book is your ally, regardless of your chosen path. (Trust me, as someone who ended up triple feeding for six months, I know firsthand there's no one-size-fits-all approach.) Whether you're planning to embrace the art of direct breastfeeding, the comfort of pumping and bottle-feeding, or a harmonious combination of both breast- and formula-feeding, you're in the right place. My mission here is not to judge or shame anyone's choices. It's to empower you with knowledge and support, no matter which route you choose to navigate. Parenthood, as you'll soon discover, is an intricate journey full of unexpected moments and personal discoveries. What works best for one family won't be the right fit for another, and that's perfectly okay. Your unique circumstances and individual choices are something to be celebrated, not critiqued.

So, rest assured that this book is here to offer guidance, insights, and a treasure trove of insider secrets, no matter how you decide to nourish and nurture your little one. Now let's embark on this adventure together, embracing the diversity of parenting paths and celebrating the shared goal of a happy, healthy baby.

The Week-by-Week Approach

I'd like to share something that would have saved me a lot of anxiety with my first baby: the "one week at a time" mindset. Instead of getting lost in the what-ifs of three months from now (like how you'll handle pumping at work or that upcoming family vacation), focus on what's happening in the next seven days. Your baby is just in their first week of life; this is your time to be present with your growing family.

Getting caught up in the what-ifs of the distant future can rob you of the joy and wonder of the present. Instead of savoring the unfolding moments with your baby, what-ifs can cloud your mind with worries and distractions. So, during the initial months of your baby's life, I encourage you to focus on taking it one week at a time. As your baby reaches around eight weeks of age, you then might begin to consider planning for two weeks at a time. Now let's explore why this mindset is a game changer, how it can ease potential anxieties, and when it might be time to chat with your healthcare provider about your feelings.

The Perks of Thinking Week by Week

1. Less Stress: Pregnancy and early motherhood bring enough changes without you trying to solve every future challenge right now. (I've seen moms trying to master latching, beginning to make a freezer milk stash, *and* trying to nurse in public all in week one. Talk about overwhelming!) Dwelling on far-off scenarios can lead to anxiety. Shifting your focus to the upcoming week simplifies your goals, making them more achievable and less anxiety-inducing.

2. Realistic Objectives: The week-by-week approach lets you be your baby's everyday superhero, tackling one challenge at a time. Instead of striving for a massive freezer full of breast milk or worrying about nursing in public several months down the line, you can focus on what matters right now—like getting comfortable with that latch or finding your feeding rhythm.

3. Increased Joy: It's easy to feel overwhelmed when thinking about the challenges that lie ahead. Allowing your mind to dwell on all the different possible scenarios can rob you of the joy of the present moment. On the other hand, focusing on the upcoming week allows you to savor the small victories and joys you experience along the way.

Rule of Thumb: Another reason to keep your focus on only the next seven days: looking too far ahead isn't just overwhelming—it can actually contribute to postpartum depression. Save tomorrow's challenges for tomorrow. Right now, you and your baby are just getting to know each other.

Special Paths: Multiples, Single Parents, and Early Arrivals

Every breastfeeding journey is unique, but some paths come with an extra special set of challenges. Whether you're preparing to feed multiples (hello, double the snuggles), navigating this journey solo, or supporting a baby who arrived a bit earlier than expected, I want you to know something: you're not alone, and yes, you can do this.

In my practice, I've supported lots of parents on these paths, and while these paths might look different from what you imagined, they're all beautiful in their own way. Let's talk about some practical strategies to help you find your flow, no matter which path you're on.

Breastfeeding Multiples

Let's talk about one of the first questions parents of multiples ask me: "How can I produce enough milk for more than one baby?" Trust me, your body is amazing and absolutely capable of this. The key is getting milk moving, either through direct breastfeeding or pumping—and sometimes both.

If both of your tiny teammates are strong feeders, you'll want them nursing as frequently as possible to build your supply. But what usually happens (and I mean *usually*) is that one baby becomes your star latcher while the other one needs some extra coaching. This is where things can get tricky—we're talking about potentially spending twenty minutes nursing one baby, another fifteen to twenty minutes bottle-feeding the other, and then still needing to pump that unused breast. Before you know it, you're looking at an hour-long production worthy of a circus juggler.

This is definitely a situation when having a professional in your corner can make all the difference. A lactation consultant can help create a game plan that works for your dynamic duo, whether that's working toward tandem feeding (nursing both babies at once) or finding a rhythm that doesn't leave you feeling like you're running a 24/7 milk café. And what if direct breastfeeding isn't working out yet? Then think of a hospital-grade double electric pump as your new best friend—aim for eight to ten pumping sessions daily to build that supply. Remember, there's no award for doing this alone, and your feeding journey is allowed to look different from what you imagined.

Single-Parent Breastfeeding

If you're navigating this journey solo, I want you to tattoo this on your heart: be kind to yourself and don't strive for perfection; instead, strive for progress. What does that look like in real life? Maybe you breastfeed half the day and then pump and bottle-feed the other half because it's quicker and lets you get better sleep. That's not failing—that's smart strategy.

Let me share some practical tips for those middle-of-the-night feeds when it's just you and baby.

> **Insider Secret:** Breast milk can stay out at room temperature (up to 77°F or 25°C) for up to 4 hours, according to the CDC and the American Academy of Pediatrics. That means you have a little flexibility before needing to run to the refrigerator at 3 A.M.

Set yourself up for success by keeping drinks and snacks near your feeding spot, and if you're pumping, have multiple sets of pump parts ready to go. That way you won't have to wash pieces in the middle of the night—because let's be real, nobody wants to be doing dishes before the sun has come up.

When it comes to building your support network, start by checking what resources your insurance provides. Many insurance plans, even health maintenance organization (HMO) plans, cover breastfeeding education and support. Get yourself a nurse advocate through your insurance and ask about available resources, including prenatal classes and doula support. And don't forget about your local WIC (Women, Infants, and Children) office—they often provide free lactation support. Your pediatrician's or obstetrician (OB)'s office can also connect you with lactation consultants and organizations that might help subsidize costs. (Remember how I said be kind to yourself? That includes asking for help.)

Early Arrivals

When your baby arrives earlier than expected, you're suddenly navigating a *very* different path than the one you planned. Breastfeeding a preterm baby comes with its own unique challenges—something I learned firsthand. Just like all babies, preterm little ones need to master the art of coordinating sucking, swallowing, and breathing, but they might need a bit more time to get there.

The main thing I want you to know? The ability to breastfeed directly often depends on your baby's ability to breathe independently. Until then, pumping becomes your superpower. Start with a hospital-grade pump and aim for twenty minutes, eight times a day. This will help establish your milk supply while your baby grows stronger. Most importantly, work with your neonatal intensive care unit (NICU)'s lactation consultant to get properly fitting pump pieces. This can make a huge difference in maximizing your milk volume, comfort, and pumping efficiency.

Here's what I tell all my preterm parents: this journey takes calm energy and patience. Your baby may be more reactive and overstimulated when there's stress and anxiety in the air. Remember, you're not on this path alone. The NICU team, including lactation consultants and sometimes feeding therapists, are there to support you.

Finding Your Flow: Every Path Is Unique

Whether your journey looks like one of these paths or follows its own unique route, remember what we talked about at the beginning of this chapter. It's about taking it one week at a time and finding what works for you and your baby (or babies). Every parent I've worked with—whether they're juggling twins, doing it solo, supporting a preterm baby, or facing other challenges—has found their flow. Sometimes it looks different than they expected (okay, it usually looks different than expected), but that's exactly why we're here: to help you discover and embrace your own path forward.

Mom-to-Mom Insight: Every baby has a different journey with breastfeeding (even with the same mother), but it is possible even if you need some support... Many people say they're "planning on breastfeeding" after having a baby, but the ones who do generally say they are "going to breastfeed." I believe the mother making a very clear decision with her intention to breastfeed plays a big part of a successful breastfeeding relationship.

—former patient Star Le

CHAPTER 3:

BUILDING YOUR MILK SQUAD DREAM TEAM

I wish I'd known...

Not everyone giving breastfeeding advice—even health-care providers—has the training to help you succeed. And scrolling through social media at 1 A.M. looking for answers... that's like trying to find your way through a maze in the dark.

Before we talk about anything else, we need to have a heart-to-heart about who you're going to turn to for help. (Because trust me, you're going to want help, and that's exactly how it should be.) Every day in my practice, I meet moms who have waited too long to get support because they were following advice from well-meaning friends, family members, or even that "expert" they found on social media who swears by some trendy breastfeeding hack.

It's important to recognize that there are plenty of well-meaning people around you who want to lend a hand. It could be your friend, sister, mom, neighbor, or even healthcare providers like your pediatrician, obstetrician, midwife, or doula. They all have your best interests at heart, and they're eager to help you on your breastfeeding journey. Now, remember that you and your journey are as unique as a fingerprint. Your birth experience, your baby, and your family all make your path a one-of-a-kind adventure, so the best breastfeeding advice isn't one-size-fits-all. Even so, there are some general rules that apply to most situations.

In this chapter, I'll cover these rules to help you navigate your support network with confidence. (Because you *are* going to be getting advice from *everyone*, including that random person at the grocery store who swears their cousin's method is foolproof.)

Rule #1: Seek Guidance from Those Who Invest Time in You

In the first weeks after birth, you and your baby need dedicated, focused support to get breastfeeding off to the best possible start. During this critical period, it's essential to have at least sixty minutes of undivided attention from a healthcare provider who is fully committed to understanding your unique situation and supporting your feeding journey. (And no, a rushed five-minute check during a pediatrician visit isn't enough. *Seriously.*)

Sixty minutes of focused time allows your provider time to observe how your body responds to your baby and assess how your baby is feeding. From there, they can offer personalized recommendations and work closely with you and your family to develop a plan tailored to your needs. They should also ensure you have a clear plan for follow-up care.

While the support of family, friends, neighbors, and doulas can be invaluable in those first few months, especially when it comes to practical help like holding the baby so you can rest or shower, it's important to remember that not everyone is a specialist in lactation and breastfeeding. Their advice, while well-intentioned, might not cover all the nuances or challenges you may encounter on your breastfeeding journey. This is where an International Board-Certified Lactation Consultant comes in. But why should you trust an IBCLC? What makes them the experts in breastfeeding?

Becoming an IBCLC requires extensive training and education focused specifically on lactation. To achieve this certification, an IBCLC must complete:

1. **Health Sciences Education:** IBCLCs must have a background in health sciences, which includes coursework in anatomy, physiology, nutrition, and other relevant fields. Many IBCLCs are also healthcare professionals, such as registered nurses, midwives, or doctors.

2. **Lactation-Specific Education:** In addition to their health sciences background, IBCLCs must complete a rigorous lactation-specific education program. This program involves more than ninety hours of study in breastfeeding management, infant and maternal health, and lactation counseling. The curriculum

covers everything from the basics of breastfeeding to complex breastfeeding challenges.

3. Clinical Experience: Before even sitting for the certification exam, aspiring IBCLCs must gain hands-on clinical experience. This involves working directly with breastfeeding families under the supervision of experienced lactation consultants. They accumulate hundreds, if not thousands, of hours assisting with breastfeeding, resolving feeding issues, and providing evidence-based care.

4. Certification Exam: After completing their education and clinical experience, candidates must pass a comprehensive certification exam administered by the International Board of Lactation Consultant Examiners (IBLCE). This exam tests their knowledge and skills in all aspects of lactation and breastfeeding support.

5. Continuing Education: Even after becoming certified, IBCLCs are required to stay current with the latest research and best practices in lactation. They must regularly complete continuing education and recertify every five years to maintain their credentials.

An IBCLC's extensive training, experience, and commitment to ongoing education make them the gold standard in breastfeeding support.[12] Think of them as your go-to expert, much like hiring a certified architect or contractor for a complex home renovation versus hiring your handy neighbor. While a handy neighbor might give you some useful DIY tips, an IBCLC has the depth of knowledge and hands-on experience needed to tackle the more intricate aspects of breastfeeding. They are the specialists who

12 IBCLC Commission, "About the IBCLC Commission," IBCLC Commission, 2022

can create a custom plan that addresses your specific needs, ensuring you have the best possible support and outcomes.

So, when you encounter challenges with breastfeeding, seeking guidance from an IBCLC is like choosing the most qualified and experienced guide to help you navigate the journey. They bring a level of expertise and dedication that goes beyond well-meaning advice, helping you and your baby build a solid foundation for a successful breastfeeding experience.

Rule #2: Rely on Expertise, Not Just Good Intentions

Here's something I wish every expecting mom knew: avoid seeking advice from someone whose knowledge is based on a handful of experiences, a few courses, or a brief certification. (You wouldn't trust someone who's taken a few contracting classes to rewire your entire house, right? So why take similar risks with your breastfeeding journey?) Find someone who has several years of hands-on, outpatient experience.

Start by researching lactation consultants in your area. Check their reviews, explore the services they offer, and find out about insurance coverage or superbill options.

> **Rule of Thumb:** Consider taking a prenatal class with a lactation consultant. You'll get a feel for their style and approach.

Feel free to call lactation consultants and ask questions to gauge their attentiveness, professionalism, and kindness.

Want to know one of my best insider tips? Reach out to like-minded postpartum moms who've been where you're headed. Ask them for lactation consultant recommendations. You'll probably hear a few names that keep coming up, giving you a great starting point for your search. It's crucial to understand that there are very few IBCLCs in private practice, and the good ones often have a waitlist. Often, mothers expect breastfeeding to come naturally, only to find out that the first few weeks bring lots of difficulties. Don't wait until your nipples are cracked and bleeding or your baby isn't gaining weight to call a lactation consultant and find out they're booked for weeks!

Make it a top priority to schedule at least one postpartum lactation consultation *before* your baby is born. So, if your due date is on June 1, then as soon as you are 34–37 weeks pregnant, you should book a postpartum lactation consultation for somewhere between June 5 and June 10. Once your baby comes, you'll be busy taking care of your little one, so take time before your baby's birth to secure an appointment with a lactation consultant and ensure that you'll have professional support.

Rule #3: Trust Your Instincts

Choosing a lactation consultant is a deeply personal decision, and it's essential to trust your instincts throughout the process. While recommendations from friends and family can be a great starting point, remember that what worked for your bestie may not necessarily be the best fit for you. The relationship between you and your lactation consultant should be one of trust, understanding, and mutual respect. As you research potential lactation consultants, pay attention to how you feel about their website, how you're treated by their receptionist, and what vibe you get from any prenatal classes they offer. (Trust me, these first impressions tell you *a lot* about their approach and whether it matches what you're looking for.) If something feels off, don't ignore that feeling—keep looking.

Chemistry and shared ideology are crucial when it comes to this relationship. You're inviting someone into one of the most intimate and challenging parts of your journey as a new parent. You should feel comfortable, supported, and confident in their ability to guide you. If you feel a connection and your values align, that's a great sign that you've found someone who will support you in the way you need. In short, don't just go with the flow or choose a consultant simply because they are covered by your insurance. Take the time to find someone who not only has the credentials and experience but also resonates with you on a personal level. Trust your instincts—they're usually trying to tell you something important.

Insider Secret: If your breastfeeding support provider says "The latch looks good, so everything is fine," even if you have pain or your baby is struggling to gain weight, find another breastfeeding support person right away!

Building Your Support Team Now

Finding the right support before your baby arrives isn't just another item on your to-do list—it's setting yourself up for success when you need it most. (And trying to find a lactation consultant in the middle of the night while dealing with painful feeds is not the time to start your research.) I see it in my practice all the time. Moms who lined up their support team before birth tend to have a smoother journey than those scrambling to find help in those emotional early days.

Remember how we talked about taking things week by week? Well, this is one time where I want you thinking ahead. Research those IBCLCs. Book that prenatal or postpartum lactation consultation now. Trust your instincts about who feels right. Because when you're in those early days of motherhood, juggling feeding sessions and trying to decode your baby's cues, you deserve to have someone in your corner who really knows their stuff—not just well-meaning advice from social media or that neighbor who breastfed three kids twenty years ago.

You're not just preparing for birth, you're preparing for those precious first weeks with your baby. Having the right support team ready to go… that's giving yourself and your baby the gift of confidence, expertise, and peace of mind. You've got this, and now you know exactly who to turn to when you need backup.

Advocating for Yourself and Your Baby

One of the most important skills you'll develop as a new mom is advocating for yourself and your baby. And let me tell you, this isn't something that comes naturally to most of us! When you're faced with medical professionals in white coats or scrubs, it can be intimidating to speak up, ask questions, or (gasp!) disagree with their recommendations. But your voice matters—especially when it comes to your breastfeeding journey.

In the hospital, don't be shy about asking for what you need. Want skin-to-skin time right after birth? Ask for it. Need help with latching during your hospital stay? You're going to need to ask for that, and you're going to need to ask both the day shift nurse and the night shift nurse to make sure it doesn't get lost in translation or during a shift change. (Because those handoffs between shifts… information absolutely gets dropped sometimes.) Be specific about what you want and need before giving birth, while you're in the hospital, and definitely before heading home.

Once you're home, this advocacy continues—and it's crucial for your breastfeeding success. Your first pediatrician checkup might be just a couple days after you get home, then at two weeks, and then at two months.

> **Rule of Thumb:** When someone gives you breastfeeding advice (even a medical professional), always ask yourself: Are they trying to understand the root cause or just offering a quick fix?

Now, what happens if your provider or consultant isn't really listening to you? Trust your gut—that's then when you need to consider getting another provider. I know this sounds harsh, but people aren't taught how to push back against medical providers because of the perceived power and authority these professionals hold. It's okay to seek a second opinion when you don't agree with your healthcare provider or consultant. (And no, you're not being "difficult" by doing this!)

At the end of the day, I want to be clear about something important: the most critical thing is that your baby must be hydrated and getting enough nutrients. It's very dangerous for a baby to not get enough milk. Not gaining weight at the appropriate intervals can lead to dehydration, seizures, and hospitalization. As long as your baby is growing appropriately, you have flexibility in your approach. But I want to be careful not to send a message that people should be digging their heels in the ground and saying, "No, I will not supplement my baby. I want to breastfeed. I'm not going to do that."

I've had that happen. The baby comes in, and their lips are dry. They have a very hoarse, dry cry. They're weak. They're lethargic. And I've had to tell the parent, "You need to go to the emergency room." I don't want that. I don't want the message being conveyed that you want to dig your heels in to the point where you're putting your baby in danger.

Instead, I want you to recognize when you're being offered what I call a "Band-Aid approach"—which isn't going to help you meet your breastfeeding goals long-term. What do I mean by that? Picture this: "Baby's not gaining weight. It's been two weeks. We're not up to birth weight yet. It's okay—just give your baby a bottle of formula." Or maybe they suggest starting to pump and bottle-feed while also breastfeeding. These quick fixes aren't getting to the root cause of what's happening.

Any solution that's not geared toward figuring out why your baby is not gaining weight or why you have a low milk supply isn't enough. If that's not the approach your provider is taking, then you need to look for a different provider who is willing to get to the root cause and do the work with you. What you want is someone who will stay alongside you, helping you investigate what's going on while still ensuring your baby is fed, but every step of the way striving to support your breastfeeding goals.

So ask yourself: Are the providers and people in your corner trying to help you figure out what's going on? Or are they just trying to push you along the conveyor belt and get you out of their clinic by offering you a quick Band-Aid fix? If nipple shields, bottles, and formula are presented as long-term solutions without additional steps to address underlying issues, then it's time to look for a different provider.

Remember, you know your body and your baby better than anyone. Advocating for thorough answers and comprehensive care isn't just your right—it's one of the most important things you can do to protect your breastfeeding journey.

Finding Your Flow: Building Your Circle of Trust

Creating a reliable support network before your baby arrives gives you a tremendous advantage in your breastfeeding journey. The professionals you choose now will become invaluable resources during those early weeks of adjustment. By researching IBCLCs, scheduling that postpartum consultation ahead of time, and trusting your instincts about who feels right for you, you're making an investment in your peace of mind.

Think of it like this: you wouldn't wait until you're standing at the base of a mountain to find your climbing guide, right? When your baby arrives and every moment feels new and sometimes overwhelming, you'll have trusted experts already in place—people whose advice you can count on without hesitation.

With your support team established and your advocacy skills ready, you'll be prepared to navigate the challenges that might come your way. You'll know when to speak up, when to ask deeper questions, and when to seek additional perspectives if something doesn't feel right. This combination of trusted support and confident self-advocacy creates a powerful foundation for your breastfeeding journey.

Rather than sorting through conflicting opinions or searching for help when you're exhausted, you'll have confidence in your carefully selected support system. This preparation allows you to focus on what truly matters: connecting with your baby and developing the rhythm that works for both of you. Knowing exactly who to call, who to trust, and how to advocate for your needs becomes a cornerstone of finding your flow in those first critical weeks.

Mom-to-Mom Insight: "While it's a natural part of your postpartum journey, breastfeeding is not always intuitive at first. I probably would have stopped breastfeeding if I didn't meet with a lactation consultant."
—former patient Celia Pennington

CHAPTER 4:

BREASTFEEDING MYTHS THAT NEED TO GO

I wish I'd known...

Many breastfeeding "rules" and myths (about pain, pacifiers, nipple confusion, spoiling babies, spicy foods) aren't based on reality and often make things harder than they need to be.

When your little one arrives, your world will shift to focus on their well-being and happiness. It's a remarkable journey, but it comes with its own set of puzzles. You might be dealing with breastfeeding discomfort, pondering the role of pacifiers, or deciding on the right formula. Every decision you make significantly impacts your baby's health and contentment. I'm here to provide answers. Think of this chapter as your myth-busting detective kit—we're going to investigate those persistent breastfeeding "rules" that keep getting passed around like neighborhood gossip and separate fact from fiction once and for all.

Myth: Pain Is Normal

You might have heard the saying "It's supposed to hurt in the beginning." Let's address this misconception straight away: breastfeeding should not be painful. When it hurts, it's a sign that something isn't quite right, which often means your baby isn't removing milk efficiently. Some mothers endure this pain, thinking it's a necessary sacrifice. I've seen countless moms in my practice white-knuckling through painful feeds because someone told them "That's just how it is." That's like continuing to drive on a flat tire because someone said bumpy rides are normal.

Here's what actually happens when you breastfeed through pain: Your little one gets hungry, you anticipate the discomfort, and as your baby tries to stimulate a milk release, your body tenses up due to pain and anxiety. This tension can actually slow your milk flow, making your baby suck harder or cry in frustration. The harder sucking causes more pain, which increases your anxiety, and the cycle continues.

Even if you manage to get your baby latched despite the pain, they're likely not transferring milk efficiently. This means they'll become hungry again sooner, leading to more frequent and still-painful nursing sessions. Over time, this pattern can lead to serious problems: low milk supply, insufficient weight gain for your baby, and even dehydration.

Working with a lactation consultant before these issues compound is crucial. They can identify what's causing the pain and help correct the latch or position to make breastfeeding comfortable and effective. You don't need to suffer through pain—in fact, doing so can undermine your breastfeeding success.

Myth: Pacifiers Will Ruin Breastfeeding

You've probably heard lots of well-meaning advice about avoiding pacifiers for the first four to six weeks to protect breastfeeding. But like most things in parenting, the reality isn't always black and white. Let's dive into the nuances so you can make the right choice for you and your baby.

Babies have a natural inclination to soothe themselves by sucking. In fact, they're born with a powerful suck reflex—anytime something touches the front part of their palate, they'll automatically start to suck. This reflex remains strong until about eight to twelve weeks of age, which is why a baby with a pacifier might seem like they never want to stop sucking.

Ideally, your little one can find comfort through latching onto your breast. However, what if latching becomes painful, or your baby gets full and frustrated because milk is coming out when all she really wants is to suck and not eat? What if your baby needs lab work and won't be able to latch during a blood draw? Or maybe your baby wails during a bath, and you can't bend over to comfort her because you're recovering from a C-section? Life throws curveballs like these, and sometimes a pacifier can be a helpful tool. The key here is to steer clear of absolute advice and avoid terms like *always* and *never*.

Now, let me share some insider insights on pacifier use. First off, many new parents don't realize that most breastfeeding newborns need to nurse frequently in the first days of life. Babies often seek to soothe themselves through sucking, which can sometimes be confused with hunger. It can be tough to differentiate between a baby who wants to comfort-suck and one who's still hungry. So I recommend limiting pacifier use to situations where your baby needs comfort during painful procedures like immunizations, circumcision, or blood draws.

A pacifier can also be useful if your baby is causing you pain or nipple damage during breastfeeding. To mimic breastfeeding, offer your baby small, frequent feeds before offering the pacifier. It's important to ensure your baby has the opportunity to eat before offering the pacifier. If you offer the pacifier before milk, your baby might spend a lot of energy using it and miss a feeding opportunity, and that's when the pacifier could negatively impact breastfeeding.

That powerful suck reflex I mentioned earlier can sometimes work against you. When a pacifier triggers this reflex, babies will suck continuously, which might make them seem satisfied when they're actually still hungry. Just remember, newborns don't lie! If they are acting hungry, they probably are. In a nutshell, when it comes to pacifiers in the early days, the key is to be mindful not to offer one when your baby genuinely needs milk instead. And remember, using a pacifier during painful procedures won't hinder breastfeeding.

Rule of Thumb: When it comes to pacifiers, think of them as a helpful tool with a specific purpose. Just like you wouldn't use a kitchen knife to tighten a screw, be intentional about when and why you're offering a pacifier. If your baby is showing hunger cues, feed first. If they need comfort during a procedure or after they're full, a pacifier can be just the right tool for the job.

Myth: Bottles Cause Nipple Confusion

Now, let's talk about a topic that can get me a little worked up: nipple confusion. First and foremost, let me emphasize this: Babies are not confused when it comes to nipples! They're actually pretty smart. However, they can develop a preference for a fast milk flow, which is where things can go off track.

It's not uncommon: you're in the hospital, and it's suggested that you supplement your baby's feeds. The staff hands you a bottle with a screw-on nipple, without any bottle-feeding instructions. (If you take a look at the nipple packaging, you will notice it's from a formula company... Ever wonder why that is?) Those hospital nipples might say "slow flow" on them, but they're designed to screw onto a ready-made bottle of formula, which can lead to your baby guzzling down the milk quickly, followed by either a deep sleep or a milk-spit-up extravaganza. Over time, your baby may end up favoring the fast flow. It should take your baby around fifteen minutes to finish a bottle-feed, regardless of the nipple type. So, you should request guidance on a technique called paced bottle-feeding, which mimics the slow release of milk from the breast. (You'll find more details in the section on paced bottle-feeding in chapter 9 and the Resources section at the end of this book).

Insider Secret: Introduce your baby to an "empty bottle" nipple for about five to six suck cycles, simulating the letdown of a breast. After that, level the bottle out parallel to the ground, allowing your baby to draw in the milk at a gentle pace. You should hear one to two sucks per swallow without significant gulping or high-pitched sounds. If you hear those large gulps and high-pitched noises, it's likely that your baby is swallowing air and drinking too quickly.

There's no such thing as nipple confusion. Babies aren't getting mixed up between breast and bottle nipples, but they can develop a preference for where the milk flows fastest. Many parents have experienced their babies rejecting the breast after a few weeks because breast milk tends to come out slower. It's not that the baby is *confused*, but instead they have a flow preference (faster).

If you want to safeguard your breastfeeding journey, invest some time in learning how to pace a bottle-feed (again, see chapter 9) and choose the right bottle nipple. Don't be fooled by the price tag. A more expensive bottle doesn't necessarily mean it's more breastfeeding-friendly. The most important factor when picking a bottle is the shape of the nipple. Look for one with a slow, gradual slope from the nipple to the base. This encourages your baby to latch widely at the base of the bottle nipple, which mimics a proper latch at the breast. On the flip side, bottles with long nipples and wide, bulbous, so-called "breast-like" shapes can lead your baby to develop poor breastfeeding habits. Your baby might latch only to the tip of the nipple, preventing them from opening their mouth and achieving a deep latch. So, steer clear of bottle marketing that claims to be breast-like. It's often just a sales pitch.

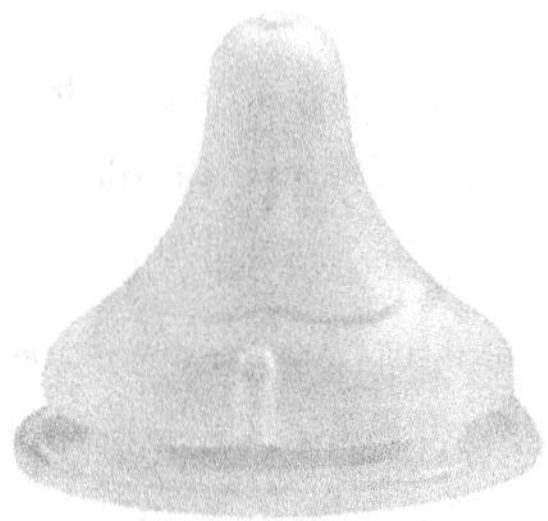

Insider Secret: Be careful not to overfeed your baby when using a bottle. Just because your baby keeps sucking on a bottle nipple after finishing a full portion of milk doesn't mean they're still hungry. Remember that automatic suck reflex we discussed? It's particularly important to be aware of the suck reflex when bottle-feeding, as babies will continue to suck and swallow even when they're full, potentially leading to overfeeding and discomfort.

Myth: You're Spoiling Your Baby

One of my greatest regrets is believing that I could spoil my baby by holding him too much. I'm not entirely certain why this notion troubled me so much. After all, when we observe nature, animals cuddle, console, and caress their offspring without any concern of overindulging them. For example, the International Primatological Society appropriately suggests that a "young monkey should not normally be separated from its mother at an early age (i.e., at 3–6 months) but should remain in contact for one year to 18 months, in most species."[13] We've all seen National Geographic shows where baby monkeys cling to their mothers all day long. These monkeys grow up just fine, and the concept of "spoiling" is a nonissue for them. Your baby spent nine months inside your

13 Viktor Reinhardt, "Artificial Weaning of Old World Monkeys: Benefits and Costs," *Animal Welfare Institute*, accessed April 3, 2025, https://awionline.org/content/artificial-weaning-old-world-monkeys-benefits-and-costs.

womb, nestled close to your heart. When they're born, they don't come with a manual on how to manipulate you. When they seem like they want to be held, it's because they want to be held. It's that simple. In my years as a lactation consultant, I've worked with thousands of babies, and I've yet to meet one with a secret agenda to manipulate their parents. Their needs are straightforward—food, comfort, connection.

In our fast-paced, industrialized world, we often substitute the essential acts of holding, nurturing, and comforting our babies with contraptions like bouncy seats and swings. These gadgets promise to do the job for us, allowing us to multitask and attend to our many other responsibilities. But it's essential to remember that originally, we were designed to birth our babies without the distractions of emails, cell phones, and televisions. These technologies didn't exist back then, and they've made us busier than ever. That's why there's a booming market for baby-holding devices like cribs that tightly swaddle and rock infants, creating white noise to try to lull them to sleep. These inventions can seem helpful, but they can't replace the magic of human touch and the unique connection between you and your baby.

While I get that these devices might be necessary now and then, especially during the first year of life, strive to be the person who offers comfort, love, and plenty of cuddles to your baby, instead of off-loading this job to an inanimate technology. I emphasize this because there's absolutely no substitute for you, Mom, or for parents in general. Yet the world will do its best to whisk your child away and immerse them in its whirlwind before you even realize it's happening. So, try your best to plan your life in a way that lets you be present for your baby and push aside the other things clamoring for your attention. These early years are what lay the foundation for the unbreakable bond you'll share with your child throughout their life. So rest assured that picking your baby up, cuddling them, and showering them with love won't ever spoil them but instead give them easy access to breastfeed!

Myth: Certain Foods in Mom's Diet Cause Gas in Babies

One of the beautiful things about breastfeeding is that you can enjoy a diverse diet while providing nourishment for your baby. The good news is that most of what you've probably heard about restricting your diet while breastfeeding is unnecessary. Spicy foods won't make your breastmilk "spicy," and if beans or broccoli make you gassy, that gas-producing effect doesn't transfer through your milk to your baby. In many cultures around the world, mothers eat diets rich in foods like beans, garlic, and spices without their babies experiencing any issues. Similarly, just because you're lactose intolerant doesn't mean your baby is.

That said, every baby is unique. While most babies aren't affected by what mom eats, a small percentage might show sensitivity to specific proteins in mom's diet. It can be very difficult to figure out what the protein sensitivity is, so you'll want to work with a professional that specializes in this. For the vast majority of breastfeeding pairs, though, there's no need to limit your culinary choices—your body does an amazing job of producing the perfect milk for your baby regardless of what's on your plate.

Now, when your infant is less than 3 months old, they might experience some gas and spit-up. This is quite common and usually not related to the foods you're eating. Instead, it's more about their developing digestive system. Several factors can contribute to your baby's gassiness and spitting up, such as overfeeding or feeding too quickly. So, if you notice your little one having these issues, it's not usually due to what you've been eating.

On the other hand, if your infant starts to develop eczema, has blood in their stool, or experiences vomiting, it's a good idea to have a conversation with their pediatrician. These symptoms could be indicative of a food sensitivity or possible food allergy. And it's usually the top allergens that are the culprits—milk, soy, eggs—not the broccoli or beans that most people worry about.[14][15] These symptoms could be linked to something else, and it's essential to keep an open line of communication with your baby's healthcare provider.

Breastfeeding is a time to savor your favorite culinary delights. Your baby benefits from a well-balanced, happy mama. Just keep in mind that those early months come with various digestive quirks for your little one, and it's usually not about what's on your plate. So eat well and enjoy these precious moments with your baby. To learn more about how your diet may affect your baby, you can check out The Boob Business Podcast episode 18[16] before your baby arrives.

Finding Your Flow: Beyond the Myths

Now that you've separated fact from fiction, you can approach your breastfeeding journey with clarity and confidence instead of confusion. Remember, these myths persist because new parents are vulnerable to well-meaning advice that promises to make things easier or better. The truth is that breastfeeding isn't about following rigid rules or believing outdated notions—it's about discovering what works for you and your baby.

---

14 American Academy of Pediatrics, "Food Allergies and Intolerances in Newborns and Infants," accessed April 3, 2025, https://www.aap.org/en/patient-care/newborn-and-infant-nutrition/food-allergies-and-intolerances-in-newborns-and-infants/.

15 Johns Hopkins Medicine, "Food Allergies in Children and Babies," last modified March 20, 2025, accessed April 3, 2025, https://www.hopkinsmedicine.org/health/conditions-and-diseases/food-allergies-in-children.

16 https://www.buzzsprout.com/1885195/episodes/11364829

As you prepare for this journey, hold onto these myth-busting insights, but also trust your instincts when something doesn't feel right. Pain isn't normal, a bottle preference isn't nipple confusion, and cuddles don't cause spoiling. Your body is designed for this incredible connection, and with accurate information replacing misconceptions, you're already on your way to finding your unique flow. The biggest breastfeeding superpower? It's not special foods or fancy techniques—it's the knowledge that allows you to make informed choices for yourself and your baby.

Mom-to-Mom Insight: "The saying that breastfeeding is natural but it doesn't come naturally is totally true."
—former patient Claudia Ochoa

CHAPTER 5:

BABY GEAR THAT ACTUALLY MATTERS

I wish I'd known...

The most expensive equipment isn't always the best, and half the "must-haves" on those baby registry checklists are completely unnecessary. The perfect bottle isn't the one with the fanciest marketing (it's the one your baby *actually* takes).

The world of baby gear... yeah, it can be a tad overwhelming. I mean, have you *seen* the baby product aisles lately? It's like a universe of gadgets and gizmos. Now, I won't hit you with an exhaustive list of every baby item out there, because, let's face it, that would be a never-ending list. Plus, with technological innovation zipping along like a speed train, anything I recommend can become outdated quickly. So instead, I'm going to give you some savvy tips to select items that can be useful while steering clear of some of the items that are purely marketing tactics.

When I was pregnant with my first, I remember wandering through Babies "R" Us countless times, obsessing over the perfect crib, stroller, car seat, and even organic cotton onesies. I scanned so many items that I wish I could get back all that time and brain power. Looking back, I spent hours researching a crib my baby wouldn't sleep in until after six months, but I didn't prepare at all for breastfeeding. I bought one set of bottles, and that was it. No pump, no nipple cream, no milk storage bags. When my milk supply struggles hit, I panic-bought products, convinced that somewhere out there was the magical device that would solve all my challenges. The truth is, I didn't know what I didn't know—I had no idea how clueless I was about what I'd actually need. Now, after helping thousands of moms navigate this same product maze, I've developed a much clearer picture of what actually helps versus what just clutters up your nursery. Let me save you from both the overwhelm and those desperate 2 A.M. online shopping sprees.

Bottles: The Lowdown

First up, bottles. Here's a golden nugget worth repeating: a higher price tag doesn't necessarily mean a better bottle. And what about those claims about special vents reducing gas? Take them with a grain of salt. Gas is more about how quickly you feed your baby and how delicate their still-developing tummies are, and there is no bottle that can replace proper bottle-feeding techniques.

You might also be wondering about those bottles that look like a breast with a super-wide base and long nipple. These bottles usually tote being "just like the breast" and "anti-colic." Don't believe the hype. You will never meet a family that says, "Using this bottle that looks like a boob really helped trick my baby into going back and forth from breast to bottle with ease." These wide-neck (or wide-base) bottles that look like boobs lack a very important quality: pliability. The silicone material is quite firm and does not easily compress and mold into the shape of an infant's mouth like a real breast does. So, instead of encouraging a deep latch, these breast-shaped bottle nipples actually encourage the infant to latch to the protruding nipple part of the bottle only, which can lead your baby to develop different oral muscles and movement patterns than are required for breastfeeding.

Now, before you fill your cart with a set of nine bottles, consider this: if you're planning to breastfeed, you might not need a fleet of bottles. Grabbing just one or two could be a smart way to start. I can't tell you how many desperate parents have come to me with a cabinet full of different bottles they've purchased, trying to find the "perfect" one their baby will accept. Save yourself that particular headache (and expense). Choose a bottle with a gentle slope (aka shoulders) and a very soft, pliable, silicone nipple. Trust me on this one—your future self will thank you when you're not staring at a mountain of rejected bottles while your baby fusses and your partner runs to the store yet again for "the bottle that might actually work this time!"

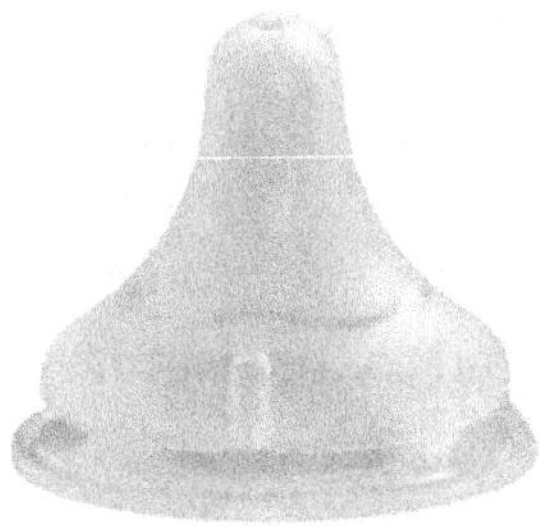

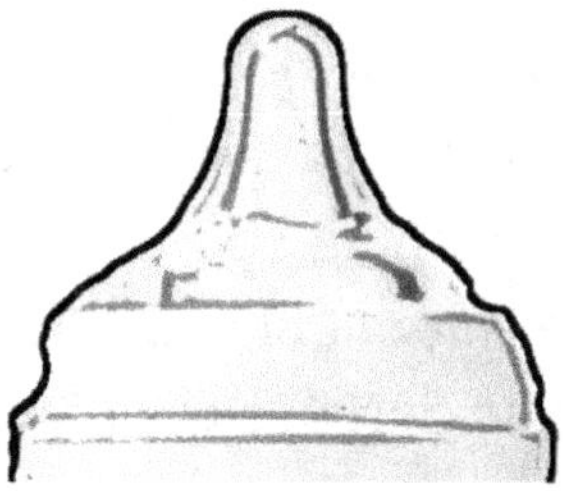

Rule of Thumb: Hold off on buying a bunch of different nipple sizes. You don't need a stash of different nipple flows. The goal should be to find a flow that best matches your breasts' flow.

Navigating Breast Pumps: Get Beyond the Fancy Marketing Hype

Breast pumps are one of the most over-marketed products in the entire baby industry (right up there with formula and baby sleep gadgets). So let me cut through all that noise and keep it simple for you: when your breastfeeding journey is just starting out, the double electric pump is your MVP. No matter what the ads say, there's no substitute for this powerhouse (except for your baby, of course). However, pump manufacturers are always tweaking their designs, so it's wise to ask your lactation consultant for a solid pump recommendation during your prenatal class or consultation.

Insider Secret: Seek pump advice from someone who is regularly hands-on with lactation patients, ideally someone caring for at least fifteen to twenty-five lactation patients monthly in an outpatient setting. While your doula, midwife, or obstetrician are fantastic, they might not have the latest insights into the pump world like a dedicated lactation professional.

Now, let's talk about those hands-free or wearable pumps. Consider them more of a sidekick than the main hero. These hands-free gadgets may not match the efficiency of the double electric wonder, meaning you might need to pump for longer to extract the same amount of milk. This might lead to those annoyingly sore nipples and perhaps even lower your milk supply.

Once your milk supply is established, stable, and doing well (after twelve to sixteen weeks postpartum), hands-free pumps can step in occasionally. Think of them as your reliable companion during a flight, commute, or special event. Some people who have an extremely robust milk supply can use wearable pumps and have no negative effects; however, I would not recommend experimenting with this if you are breastfeeding your first child and you are making just enough milk for your baby. Ultimately, it's all about balance. Stick with the double electric pump in the beginning, and once things are steady, then you can bring in the hands-free sidekick for occasional pumping sessions.

> **Rule of Thumb:** Don't rely on hands-free or portable pumps until after at least the first twelve weeks of life.

Choosing the Right Flange Size

A flange is the funnel-shaped part of the breast pump that goes over the nipple to extract milk. Pumps often come with just two flange sizes: 24 mm and 28 mm. Most women, however, fall into the 15–19 mm range, which is quite different from those standard sizes. Now, let that sink in. It's like trying to buy shoes and only finding two pairs that are three sizes too big. Imagine strolling around Disney World in oversized shoes. The result? Sore feet, blisters, and the potential for damage to your feet, ankles, and shins.

Using flanges that are too big is a bit like wearing those oversized shoes. It can lead to reduced milk output, discomfort, and even tissue damage to the breast and nipple. In the world of pump flanges, bigger is not better. So let's avoid the pitfalls of the one-size-fits-all approach. Work with an experienced lactation consultant to help find the flange size that's just right for you. It's not just about comfort—it's about optimizing your pumping experience for better milk output and overall breast health. Your lactation consultant can guide you in selecting the right size, helping ensure your pumping journey is comfortable and effective.

Pumping Bras

If you plan to pump, having a properly fitted pumping bra can be very helpful. Often after birth, your wrists and fingers can ache for a few weeks; this can be caused by a change in hormones and the new repetitive movements of holding your baby[17]. Having your hands free when pumping can make a world of difference. I recommend waiting until after you deliver your baby to try on pumping bras. You will be amazed at how much your breasts can grow from thirty-four weeks of pregnancy to two weeks postpartum. So, to avoid a too-tight bra, plan to purchase a pumping bra during the postpartum period.

> **Insider Secret:** Stay away from strapless pumping bras. They can act like a tourniquet to your milk flow and cause additional complications such as inflammation to the breast tissue. Instead, opt for a pumping bra with typical shoulder straps.

17 American Journal of Roentgenology (AJR), "De Quervain's Tenosynovitis: Postpartum Wrist Pain in New Mothers," AJR, 2020.

Nonessential Equipment

When it comes to preparing for your breastfeeding journey, it's important to distinguish between essential items and those that might be marketed as necessary but aren't truly required for successful breastfeeding. There are entire store aisles dedicated to products that claim to "revolutionize" your experience, but let me be real with you—most will just collect dust while emptying your wallet. Think of me as your shopping bodyguard here, steering you away from the fancy marketing and toward what actually matters. Here's my honest guide to what you can confidently skip without a second thought (aka they're generally nonessential):

1. **Breast Massager:** While some breastfeeding parents find massagers helpful for relieving discomfort or promoting milk flow, they are not necessary for everyone and can sometimes cause harm. You can often massage your breasts more gently using your hands, and you may find that simple techniques like hand expression or warm compresses are sufficient.

2. **Special Baby Containers, Swings, Vibrating/Rocking Cribs, and Sleep Aids That Tightly Restrict Your Baby's Arms:** These items can be helpful for soothing or entertaining your baby in the short term, but they are not necessary and can sometimes interfere with important protective, primitive reflexes.

Instead of investing in fancy gadgets that restrict your baby's movement, consider the original hands-free solution: babywearing. I'm a huge fan of good carriers and wraps that keep your little one close. Babywearing, the practice of carrying your baby close to your body using a carrier or sling, offers numerous benefits for both the parent and child. Not only does it provide a convenient way to keep your baby close while having your hands free for other tasks, but it also promotes strong parent-infant attachment.

Babies who are carried often experience reduced crying and fussiness, improved emotional regulation, and enhanced physical development.[18]

What's more, babywearing is actually beneficial for your breastfeeding journey. The close proximity of your baby stimulates the release of oxytocin, the hormone responsible for milk release, which can help support breastfeeding success. Additionally, babywearing allows for easy and discreet nursing on the go, making it simpler for you to respond to your baby's feeding cues no matter where you are.

3. Special Soap to Clean Bottles and Pump Parts: While it's important to keep your bottles and pump parts clean, you don't necessarily need to purchase special soap for this purpose. Mild dish soap or even boiling water are often sufficient for cleaning these items effectively. Save yourself some money by skipping the specialized cleaning products and opting for soap that you currently use to wash your dishes instead.

Finding Your Flow: Gear Without the Gimmicks

By focusing on the essentials and avoiding unnecessary gadgets or products, you can streamline your breastfeeding journey and avoid getting bogged down by unnecessary clutter (not to mention save yourself a small fortune!). Remember, every parent and baby is different, so what works for one family may not work for another. The Instagram-perfect nursery filled with every gadget under the sun doesn't equal breastfeeding success—your confidence and comfort do. Trust your instincts, prioritize items that truly support your breastfeeding goals, and remember that

---

18 Academic Journal of Pediatrics & Neonatology (AJPN), "Babywearing Practices and Effects on Parental, Child Physical and Emotional Outcomes," AJPN, June 6, 2022.

you're already equipped with the most important tools: your beautiful mama instincts and those amazing milk-making breasts!

> **Mom-to-Mom Insight:** "Finding the right pump and pump equipment is like finding the perfect bra. Sometimes not every pump may work the same way it would for others, nor will everyone's flange size be the same. It takes trial and error and getting with a great lactation consultant, like Naiomi. It took me three different flange sizes to find the perfect fit. Now I'm confident in breastfeeding and pumping, and I'm proud to say my journey isn't over!"
> —former patient Kalie Karl

PART II:

WHAT I WISH I'D KNOWN IN THE FIRST DAYS

CHAPTER 6:

FIRST FEEDS WITHOUT FEAR

I wish I'd known...

Watch the baby, not the clock. Trying to schedule your baby to eat every three hours in the early weeks is just asking for anxiety. Breastfed babies want you to watch them for hunger cues, not the clock.

Ah, the thrilling debut of your baby's life! These first days are filled with precious moments of awe and exploration and (let's be honest) a lot of "Hmm... what do I do now?" moments too. As you cradle your newborn for the very first time, emotions swirl within you like a perfectly chaotic snow globe of joy, wonder, and uncertainty.

When my first son arrived earlier than expected, my experience was nothing like the peaceful "golden hours" I wish I'd had. The "golden hours" refer to those first one to two crucial hours right after birth—a special window when your baby is naturally alert and ready to begin breastfeeding before falling into a deep sleep that can last up to 24 hours. During this brief but magical time, babies are typically awake and responsive, often licking, mouthing, and even doing a little "breast crawl" to find the nipple on their own. This skin-to-skin contact and first latch, even if brief, helps your baby imprint and sets the foundation for successful breastfeeding when they wake up again.

But my introduction to motherhood looked very different. I was young, in pain (due to an episiotomy and an epidural that didn't work), and completely unprepared. I had no idea what colostrum even was, let alone its importance (more on this in a moment). With my baby being premature and jaundiced, those early feeding attempts were filled with anxiety rather than magic. I remember looking at his tiny face and thinking, Am I doing this right? Is he getting anything at all? No one explained that his constant hunger and my seemingly empty breasts were actually part of a normal pattern for a preterm baby. Instead, I felt like I was failing from the very start.

That's exactly why I'm so passionate about helping you have a different experience. What I went through doesn't have to be your story. With the right information and support, these first moments with your baby can be what they're meant to be: precious, connected, and, yes, even magical.

This chapter is your insider's guide to those crucial first feeds. Think of the golden hours as your front-row seat to one of the most captivating shows on Earth—and let me tell you, when you know what to expect, it truly is pure magic.

What to Expect During the Golden Hours

Okay, let's talk about what really happens in those first magical hours (not the polished Instagram version, but the real deal). Because trust me, knowing what to expect makes all the difference between thinking *Is this normal?* and confidently enjoying this once-in-a-lifetime moment.

Imagine your newborn baby, nestled against your chest, instinctively seeking comfort and nourishment from your breast. This beautiful moment isn't just about hunger or soothing—it's about a profound connection forged through the powerful process of imprinting. Newborn mammals, including humans, can recognize their mothers, primarily through touch and taste. This innate ability, known as imprinting, is nature's way of ensuring that babies bond with their mothers and find the source of life-sustaining nourishment: the breast.[19]

During imprinting, your baby's delicate mouth explores the world, searching for the unique features of your nipple. This isn't just random suckling—it's a genetically programmed behavior designed to help your baby latch onto the breast, initiate

19 PubMed Central, "Neonatal Sensory Recognition and Oral Tactile Imprinting in Human Newborns," PubMed Central, 2021.

breastfeeding, and create a deep, unbreakable bond with you. However, this precious process can be disrupted. When babies engage in nonnutritive sucking on bottles or pacifiers, they may miss out on the vital stimulation needed to support breastfeeding. Studies have shown that babies who rely on pacifiers during this early period in their life may breastfeed for shorter durations, highlighting the importance of understanding and supporting the natural imprinting process.[20]

So, as you prepare to welcome your little one into the world, remember the magic of imprinting. Embrace those tender moments of skin-to-skin contact and let your baby's instinctive search for your breast be a testament to the deep bond you are developing. In these fleeting moments, it's tempting to let the outside world creep in. Racing thoughts, doubts, worries, and fears might whisper in your ear, threatening to steal the joy from these irreplaceable early moments. However, I encourage you to hold them at bay, for these minutes are precious and limited. In a world that rarely slows down, this is your chance to pause and revel in the extraordinary. Let those distractions and fears melt away as you embrace the wonder of your new baby.

The Deep-Sleep Phase: A Worn-Out Mama and Baby

Now, following their initial exploratory amazement at the world, most newborns expertly transition into the next phase, which experts refer to as the deep-sleep phase. Think of it as their power nap session, a crucial time for them to conserve energy and facilitate growth. It's also your golden opportunity to indulge in some well-deserved rest and rejuvenation.

---

20 PubMed, "Early Pacifier Use and Its Impact on Breastfeeding Duration," PubMed, 2013.

As your baby peacefully slumbers in this phase, you can prioritize self-care, catch up on some much-needed sleep, or even treat yourself to a snack. You've certainly earned it! Childbirth is undoubtedly a challenging experience, and looking after your own well-being is paramount for both you and your precious bundle. Now, while it might be tempting to scroll through your phone or engage in social media, consider giving yourself a break from screens. Take this moment to be present, enjoy a nourishing meal, and simply unwind. And while both you and your baby rest, your body continues its remarkable work, preparing that precious early milk your baby will need when they wake.

> **Insider Secret:** Babies are more likely to open their eyes in environments with softer, dimmer lighting. So if you want to see their eyes in their first hours of life, dim the lights a bit.

Colostrum and Its Nutritional Value: Nature's First Meal After the Deep Sleep

While you were busy preparing for your baby's arrival (and maybe obsessing over nursery colors like I did), your body was already quietly working its magic behind the scenes.

Way back in the second trimester, around the twentieth week of your pregnancy, it quietly started crafting something truly special: colostrum, the "liquid gold" for your baby's health journey.[21] Colostrum is the first "milk" your body makes. It's not just rich in nutrients—it's basically a superhero potion for your baby's tummy and immune system.[22] Think of colostrum as a blend of the finest superfoods, a nutritional powerhouse that gives your little one

21 Pregnancy Birth and Baby, "Antenatal Expression of Colostrum," Healthdirect Australia, April 2025.

22 MedicalXpress, "Colostrum Provides Long-Lasting Immunity Boost for Babies," February 14, 2024.

everything they need during those crucial early days. Even though there's not a lot of it in terms of volume, the value of colostrum is immeasurable, as it sets your baby on the path to optimal health. But here's the truly fascinating part: colostrum also acts like a guardian of your baby's tummy. It has this unique ability to line your baby's gut with protective elements. The colostrum strengthens your baby's gut, making it less welcoming to harmful microorganisms. It's nature's way of ensuring your little one's safety in this new and sometimes unpredictable world.

How Much Milk Does Your Baby Need?

Understanding your baby's feeding needs during their first day of life is essential. Generally speaking, your newborn will need about 40–60 milliliters of colostrum during their first twenty-four hours of life,[23] which is equivalent to 8–12 teaspoons total. On days two and three, your newborn will need about 170–220 milliliters in a twenty-four-hour period,[24] which is equivalent to 5.75–7.5 ounces total.

I know what you're thinking—that doesn't sound like much! But your baby has a tiny tummy (more on just how tiny in a moment). And that's exactly why those small amounts are perfect. It's like nature's portion control at its finest.

How Big Is Their Tummy?

In the first hours of life, your baby's tummy is not much larger than a cherry or a marble,[25] but it's designed perfectly for the precious drops of colostrum you'll provide during those initial feeds. This tiny tummy is like a canvas awaiting the first brushstrokes of a masterpiece, gradually growing and adapting over the first few days to accommodate larger milk volumes as your mature milk arrives. By day two or three, it will have expanded to roughly the

23 NHS, "Breastfeeding: The First Few Days," NHS, 2025.

24 Health Service Executive (HSE), "How Much Breast Milk to Express," HSE.ie, 2025.

25 La Leche League Canada, "Newborns Have Small Stomachs," January 1, 2022.

size of a plump strawberry.[26] So, in these early hours, it's not about filling that little tummy up to capacity. It's about nurturing it with the liquid gold of colostrum. Think of it like this: you wouldn't pour a gallon of water into a shot glass, right? Your baby's tummy works the same way. Those tiny drops of colostrum are exactly the right serving size.

But here's a little secret they don't always tell you: despite this tiny tummy, if you were to offer your baby a bottle with around 1–1.5 ounces of breast milk on their very first day of life, they might drink it down with fervor and continue to suck as if they're craving more. It's a moment that often leaves new parents second-guessing their feeding plan, contemplating whether their breasts are producing enough colostrum to satiate their little one's appetite. But there's no need to worry.

So why do they continue to suck? Well, as we discussed earlier, babies have this incredible reflex that's like a "suck button." When anything touches the front part of the roof of their mouth, called the hard palate, it's like flipping a switch, and they start to suck. It's their way of saying, "Hey, what's this?"—not necessarily a cry for immediate hunger. So, when your baby shows enthusiasm for sucking, there's no need to fret. In fact, you should welcome it.

During this early phase of their life, it's smart to offer them small, frequent feedings. This strategy not only protects your breastfeeding journey from being sabotaged by supplementation that may not be needed but also keeps issues like overfeeding (which can happen whether you're using the breast or a bottle) and tummy discomfort, like spit-up or reflux, at bay.

26 BabyCentre UK, "How Big Is Your Baby's Stomach: Photos," March 20, 2024.

Rule of Thumb: For a visual guide on how much milk or colostrum to offer your baby, go to the Resources section.

How Often Do They Need to Eat?

In the first twenty-four to forty-eight hours after birth, your baby's feeding needs can vary. Some newborns may latch and feed frequently, like twelve times per day, while others may feed less often, like closer to eight times per day. Here's where you need to ditch the clock and tune into your baby's signals instead. Your baby doesn't care what time it is—they care about when they're hungry. And learning to read those cues? That's your new superpower. They will display signs of readiness to feed, such as rooting, licking their lips, or bringing their hands to their mouth.

It's crucial to remember that babies don't lie. If they seem hungry, they probably are. It's common for mothers to be surprised by how frequently their baby wants to eat during the first week or two of life. Instead of offering a feeding when the baby signals hunger, some parents opt for a pacifier. The result? The baby spends about fifteen minutes sucking on the pacifier, gets rocked to sleep, and ends up missing a feeding opportunity. After about thirty minutes, they wake up crying and clearly showing signs of hunger. But crying is a late sign of hunger in babies. Your baby hasn't quite figured out that you won't let them go hungry. So when they start feeling hungry, it's like a tiny internal alarm going off, saying, "Feed me now, or I might starve!"

Rule of Thumb: It is not recommended to attempt putting a newborn on a schedule that would encourage the caregiver to stretch feeds out despite the newborn showing signs of hunger. The first few months of life are *not* the time to try to put your baby on a strict feeding schedule. It can be harmful to their metabolism, growth, and development.

Waiting until your baby is very hungry often leads to a frustrated and possibly even combative latching experience. Instead of waiting for your newborn to get super hungry, it's a great idea to feed them frequently in shorter sessions. During the first week after birth, aim for about ten to fifteen minutes on each side. You might need to gently wake your baby after the first side or let them rest and digest for ten to twenty minutes before offering the second side. This feeding method is sometimes playfully referred to as "Dinner Then Dessert."

Rule of Thumb: Feeding fifteen minutes on each breast may not be best practice after the first week of life. You and your lactation consultant will need to assess your milk supply and your baby's ability to remove milk in order to determine how long to offer each breast as your baby grows.

The key here is to listen for swallowing sounds. The minutes your baby spends at the breast matter less than the time they actively suck and swallow. Working with a lactation consultant to understand your baby's unique suck-swallow patterns can be incredibly helpful in teaching both you and your baby how to breastfeed efficiently.

Reading Your Baby's Feeding Cues

Figuring out if your baby is getting enough colostrum in those first twenty-four to forty-eight hours can feel like trying to solve a Rubik's Cube while sleep-deprived. You're equipped with the world's best milk, but how do you know it's reaching your little one effectively?

First, let's clear up a common misconception: the amount of time your baby spends at the breast isn't necessarily proportional to how much milk or colostrum they're receiving. In these initial days, your baby might appear to be dozing off or pausing frequently during feeds, which can understandably make you question whether they're getting enough nourishment. Therefore, it's important to recognize the signs of active and efficient feeds. Active nursing, or active milk transfer, typically involves your baby sucking one to three times, followed by swallowing. Brief pauses, lasting two to five seconds, are normal during a feed. However, if your baby is pausing more frequently or for extended periods, the nursing session may be becoming inefficient.

In such cases, your baby might be more interested in napping than eating. This situation is common and not anyone's fault. There are various reasons why newborns become sleepy at the breast. Some of these reasons are related to medical factors, which we'll explore in later chapters.

Insider Secret: Compressing your breast while breastfeeding can significantly increase the amount of milk and number of calories your baby gets.

How to Tell If They Are Getting Enough to Eat

Now, let's talk about the subtle cues that can help you gauge whether your baby is getting enough to eat. During these early days, robust swallowing sounds might not be immediately evident because your body is producing colostrum, not yet the larger volumes of milk that typically start appearing around day three to five after birth.

Here are some reassuring signs to look for:

1. **Calm and Relaxation During Feeds:** Your baby should seem relaxed during feeds, not overly fussy or frustrated.

2. **Self-Detachment:** Your baby should come off the breast on their own when they're finished, showing a sense of satiety.

3. **Moist Mouth:** After feeds, check your baby's mouth. It should appear moist, indicating they've been effectively feeding.

4. **Contentment After Feeds:** A well-fed baby appears satisfied after most feeds, displaying a sense of comfort.

Weight is another factor to consider. It is normal for newborns to lose some weight during their initial days. However, this weight loss should not exceed 8–10 percent of their birth weight. By the fourth day of life, your baby should stop losing weight and begin gaining weight at an average rate of about 1 ounce per day.[27] Precise measurements can be challenging with standard baby or home scales due to the small increments involved, so I highly recommend scheduling an evaluation with a lactation consultant who has the proper equipment during your baby's first week of life. They can provide invaluable insights and support to

27 Stanford Medicine, "Infant with Loss of 10% Birth Weight," Stanford Medicine, 2024.

ensure your baby is on the right track in this crucial early phase of breastfeeding.

How Many Wet and Dirty Diapers Should They Have?

One of the indicators that your baby is getting enough colostrum and staying adequately hydrated is their diaper output. On the first day of life, you can expect at least one wet diaper and one dirty diaper. However, as your baby progresses through the first twenty-four hours, you should aim for at least two wet diapers at two days old, three wet diapers at three days old, and so on until there are more than five wet diapers and several stooled diapers per day. This is a terrific sign of good feeding and hydration.

Rule of Thumb: It is extremely easy to "miss" a pee because disposable diapers are so absorbent nowadays. To ensure you don't miss a pee, place a sheet of toilet paper in the diaper. If the toilet paper is wet when you open the diaper, then your baby peed! If you wait to see the blue line that is promised to appear in some diapers when wet, you may actually have two to three pees in the diaper by then.

Finding Your Flow: Embracing These Precious Early Days

These first feeding days might feel like a blur, but they're setting the foundation for everything that follows. Remember when we talked about taking things one week at a time? Even one day at a time? This is exactly why. These early moments aren't about perfection—they're about connection, learning, and trusting the process.

What I wish someone had told me with my first baby is that every tiny drop of colostrum, every sleepy feed, every moment spent skin-to-skin is building something incredible between you and your baby. You're feeding your little one *and* you're sending powerful signals to your body about what comes next.

And what comes next? That's when your body really kicks into high gear. In the coming chapter, we'll dive into exactly how your milk supply builds and how you can support it like the milk-making boss you were born to be. With the right information and support (the kind I wish I'd had from the beginning), you'll be amazed at what you and your baby can accomplish together.

> **Mom-to-Mom Insight:** "Breastfeeding is one of the hardest and most rewarding things I've ever done. It's an incredibly individualized experience between each baby and mom. Be confident in your choices, and don't let others dictate what is 'best' for your family."
> —former patient C.R.

CHAPTER 7:

POWER MOVES FOR MAXIMUM MILK SUPPLY

I wish I'd known...

Your boobs are like smart devices that need proper setup. Configure them correctly in the first week, and they'll deliver milk on demand without constant troubleshooting. Skip the initial programming, and you'll be dealing with "error messages" and "system resets" for months.

The First Days: Setting the Lactation Thermostat

I wish someone had told me that what I did in those very first days would set the tone for my entire milk production journey. I was so focused on the immediate challenges that I had no idea I was actually programming my body's milk-making capacity. Specifically, I wish I'd known that starting milk removal within the first two hours after birth and then continuing with at least eight feedings every twenty-four hours is crucial for maximizing long-term milk supply.

Despite the overwhelming exhaustion of those early days, those frequent and effective milk removals (hopefully by your baby) are essential programming steps. I also wish someone had emphasized that even when I felt like I could barely keep my eyes open, maintaining those eight-plus breastfeeding or pumping sessions daily was setting the foundation for my future milk production. It wasn't until years later, when I became a lactation consultant, that I understood how those early days work like setting a thermostat for your milk supply. This knowledge completely changed how I support new moms today.

When I talk about setting up your milk supply for success, I'm often met with anxious questions about production. Almost every new mom worries about having enough milk. You've probably seen those social media pics of freezers stacked with pumped milk and wondered, *Is that what I need to aim for?* Well, let me clear things up right away: you don't need a massive milk stash. Seriously, don't stress about filling a deep freezer to the brim. That's not what this is about! Instead, I suggest that you take it one week at a time (remember our mantra from chapter 2?) and focus on filling your baby instead of the freezer for right now.

There's no need to get caught up in thinking about how many ounces you'll need when you head back to work or for that epic annual girls' trip (although that does sound fantastic, doesn't it?). Let's just focus on the next seven days. Again, what you do during those initial days following childbirth are the most important factors to influence long-term milk production. These first few days are like programming an internal "lactation thermostat" that is rather particular and needy.

Skipping this "programming" step can result in lower long-term milk production abilities. So if you want to supercharge your milk supply in the long run, it's all about laying the right foundation from the very beginning. Your body is most receptive to these cues in the first week post-birth, making it the perfect time to establish a robust milk supply that will meet your baby's growing needs.

Practical Strategies for Success

Let me break down some practical strategies that I wish someone had handed me on a silver platter during that first week:

1. Focus on Frequent and Effective Milk Removal: Your baby's tummy is small, but their appetite for colostrum is colossal. Feed them whenever they show signs of hunger, and don't worry if it seems like they're nursing around the clock—it's perfectly normal. Frequent and thorough milk removal during the first two weeks is your golden ticket to a bountiful supply.

2. Express by Hand: In addition to nursing, consider hand expression. This technique allows you to express (*express* is just a fancy term that means manually extracting milk from the breasts) precious drops of colostrum, which can be fed to your baby even if they're having trouble latching. It's a fantastic way to ensure no drop goes to waste.

I know, I know—hand expression sounds so old-school when there are fancy pumps everywhere. But trust me on this one. When my milk was just coming in, my hands were way more effective than any pump. There's something about that skin-to-skin contact and gentle pressure that just works magic in those early days.

Insider Secret: Be sure to visit firstdroplets.com, a fantastic website dedicated to teaching you all about hand-expression techniques and feeding your baby during the first few days of life.

Rule of Thumb: In the early days when you're producing colostrum, hand express directly into a spoon or container rather than using a pump. This prevents precious drops from getting stuck in pump parts and ensures your baby gets every bit of this liquid gold.

3. Stay Hydrated and Well-Nourished: Remember to take care of yourself. Drink plenty of sugar-free fluids and maintain a nutrient-dense diet. You will know you are properly hydrated when your urine is pale yellow (like watered-down lemonade). Your body needs those nutrients and hydration to produce milk. Please note that overhydrating is not helpful.

4. Prioritize Skin-to-Skin Contact: Practice skin-to-skin contact as often as possible. This close bonding time helps regulate your baby's body temperature and blood sugar,[28] and it encourages them to feed more effectively.

28 Sanford Health, "The 'Golden Hour': Giving Your Newborn the Best Start," September 26, 2022.

5. Get Comfortable: Ensure that both you and your baby are comfortable during feedings. Use pillows or a nursing cushion to support your body and make sure your baby has a good latch.

6. Trust Your Instincts: If something doesn't feel right, trust your instincts and seek support. A lactation consultant, your healthcare provider, or a support group can offer guidance and reassurance. As I mentioned earlier, I strongly recommend scheduling an appointment with a lactation consultant before you leave the hospital. Just call them up and book an appointment for five to seven days after the birth of your baby.

7. Rest and Recover: Rest is essential for both you and your baby. Try to catch some z's when your baby is sleeping to aid your recovery and overall well-being.

8. Be Patient: Building a robust milk supply takes time, and every baby is unique. Be patient with yourself and your little one, and remember that breastfeeding is a learning experience for both of you.

9. Do Not Tolerate Pain: I want you to remember this rule! If the latch hurts, then your baby is not transferring milk effectively. Trying to power through the pain does not help anyone. This is one I learned the hard way, and I see moms struggling with it every day in my practice. We're taught to "push through the pain" in so many areas of life, but breastfeeding shouldn't be one of them. Pain is your body's way of saying, "Hey, something's not right here!" So listen to it, okay? And then get help from a lactation consultant until you can achieve a pain-free latch.

In a nutshell, the first week of your breastfeeding journey lays the foundation for a successful milk supply. By focusing on this crucial period and implementing these practical strategies, you're setting yourself up for a fulfilling and nourishing experience that benefits both you and your precious baby. So, embrace the journey, stay positive, be quick to get help, and relish those beautiful moments of bonding with your little one.

If you or your baby require more intensive medical care after birth, the plan to protect your milk supply will look a little different. We will cover more details in chapters 13 and 14.

Factors That Can Influence Milk Production

In the early days and weeks after giving birth, establishing a healthy milk supply is a top priority for many new mothers. Let's get real about what actually impacts your milk-making abilities. (Spoiler alert: it's not those lactation cookies that keep popping up in your social media feed!)

While milk production is a natural process, several factors can influence it. Let's talk about food first. What you eat doesn't typically affect how much milk you make, but it can influence the quality of fat in your breast milk. Your amazing body will produce milk with similar levels of calories, carbohydrates, and protein regardless of your diet, but the type of fats in your milk will reflect the fats you consume. Eating foods rich in healthy fats like avocados, walnuts, olive oil, and salmon provides higher quality fats than those from highly processed foods.

This is why a balanced diet matters for breastfeeding—not because you need special "milk-boosting" foods, but because quality nutrition supports both your milk and your overall health. Be skeptical of marketing that promotes special cookies and bars claiming to increase milk supply. Instead, focus on nutrient-dense whole foods and staying well-hydrated throughout the day. Your body is already designed to make the perfect amount of milk for your baby; your diet just helps ensure it's the best quality it can be.

Next, hormones play a significant role. During pregnancy, your body undergoes hormonal changes to prepare for breastfeeding. After giving birth, hormone levels fluctuate, sending signals to your body to start producing milk. However, hormonal imbalances, such as those associated with thyroid disease or diabetes, can affect milk production.[29] If you have any underlying health conditions or concerns about hormonal imbalances, it's essential to discuss them with your healthcare provider.

Additionally, the postpartum period can be both physically and emotionally challenging, and stress levels can affect your body's ability to produce milk. Finding ways to manage stress, such as practicing relaxation techniques, getting enough rest, and seeking support from loved ones, can help support milk production.

Women in their mid- to late-thirties, as well as those who have experienced infertility or metabolic disorders such as thyroid disease or diabetes, may find it beneficial to work with a functional health provider. These healthcare professionals take a holistic approach to health by addressing underlying issues that may impact fertility and breastfeeding, such as hormonal imbalances or metabolic disorders. By addressing these concerns early on, you can optimize your chances of successful breastfeeding and better ensure the health and well-being of both you and your baby.

29 PubMed Central, "Do Thyroid Diseases During Pregnancy and Lactation Affect Milk Production?" November 30, 2020.

Finding Your Flow: Abundance Without Anxiety

All these factors—diet, hormones, stress levels—combine to create your unique breastfeeding experience. While professional support can be incredibly valuable (especially if you have specific health concerns), understanding how to set your body up for milk-making success from day one is what matters most.

Remember how I mentioned my triple-feeding marathon in the introduction? That wasn't fun for anyone (not for me and certainly not for my baby). But here's what I've learned since then: when you implement the strategies we've discussed in this chapter, you're much less likely to end up in that exhausting cycle. You deserve to enjoy these early weeks with your baby, not spend them stressing about every drop of milk. So take these approaches, make them your own, and know that you're laying the groundwork for a breastfeeding journey that works for both you and your little one. You've got this!

Mom-to-Mom Insight: "I wish I had known that even though I would have a low supply, there were ways I could increase it. I also wish I had known that the amount I was able to produce wasn't reflective of my value as a mother and that even my small supply was helpful for my daughter."
—former patient Caroline Seikel

CHAPTER 8:

COOL MOVES FOR NAVIGATING ENGORGEMENT

I wish I'd known...

When your breasts are engorged, the last thing you want to do is fight them into submission. Those rock-hard boobs need gentle care—think how you'd pet a kitten, not how you'd give a deep-tissue massage. The harder you attack the swelling, the worse it can get.

Amid the joy and wonder of welcoming your newborn into the world, your body is also undergoing significant changes, including the preparation for and arrival of milk for your little one.

Let me paint a picture of what typically happens: Somewhere between day three and day five after giving birth, you'll wake up one morning and your breasts will suddenly feel like rocks—definitely a lot firmer than they were just twenty-four hours earlier. They might feel hot, heavy, stiff, and more tender to the touch than usual. Your first thought will probably be, *Wow, my milk came in!* followed quickly by, *What the heck do I do with this?!*

Here's where most moms get confused. Most people think their breasts are full with milk, but that's actually a myth. What's really happening is that your body, which has been carrying all that extra fluid to support your pregnancy, is now redirecting some of that fluid to your breast tissue. While this transition is a marvel of nature, it can sometimes lead to a temporary challenge known as engorgement.

Understanding Engorgement: The Science Behind the Swelling

Let's dig a little deeper into what's actually happening in your body, because there's a lot of confusion out there. And trust me, when your breasts feel like they might explode, the last thing you need is confusing advice from well-meaning friends or random internet searches.

What most people don't realize is that engorgement isn't primarily about milk volume. The real culprit is edema—medical speak for swelling caused by excess fluid trapped in your tissue. It's basically your pregnancy fluid finding a new home in your breast tissue. Yes, there's an increase in milk production happening simultaneously, but it's the combination of these factors that creates that uncomfortable rock-hard feeling.

So what doesn't work? This is important: pumping typically doesn't improve engorgement. I know it *seems* logical—if your breasts feel full, empty them, right? But pumping can actually cause more edema and swelling in your breast tissue and yield little to no milk removal. And those aggressive massage techniques you might see recommended online? They can make things worse by damaging delicate breast tissue and increasing inflammation and swelling.

I know—when you're in pain, you want to *do* something to fix it. But sometimes less truly is more. The approaches I'm going to share might seem too simple, but they're backed by research, and, more importantly, they actually work!

The Gentle and Evidence-Based Approach to Managing Engorgement

Here's a tool kit of evidence-based interventions for managing engorgement while your body adjusts to its new role as a milk-making machine (I didn't invent these approaches—I'm sharing what research has shown to be most effective):

1. Maintain a Normal Feeding or Pumping Schedule: Contrary to the outdated belief that you must "fully drain" your breasts frequently, adhere to your baby's natural feeding rhythm. Feeding on demand allows your body to produce milk at a pace that aligns with your baby's requirements. There is no need to pump to empty—or pump at all, for that matter, if your baby is removing milk from you.

Rule of Thumb: Your hands are going to be more effective than a pump when managing engorgement. And what I mean by *hands* is learning hand expression, gentle lymphatic drainage, or reverse pressure softening. See the Resources section for more information.

2. **Embrace Ice or Cold Packs:** Applying ice or cold packs to your breasts for fifteen to twenty minutes can provide relief by reducing inflammation and swelling. Be sure to wrap the ice pack in a thin cloth or towel to protect your skin.

3. **Wear a Comfortable, Supportive Bra:** Choose a well-fitting, supportive bra that doesn't constrict or compress your breasts. The goal is to provide comfort while avoiding additional pressure.

4. **Use Gentle Touch:** Treat your breasts with the tenderness reserved for petting a cat. Steer clear of vigorous, deep massaging or pressing, as these actions may exacerbate engorgement. Instead, use gentle fingertip touches to guide excess fluid toward your armpit, where your lymphatic system can assist in alleviating the pressure. *Gentle* is the name of the game here.

5. **Consider Medications for Pain Relief:** If you find yourself struggling with discomfort, discuss the use of acetaminophen or ibuprofen with your primary care provider (PCP). These medications can help reduce swelling and provide pain relief.

6. **Monitor and Consult:** Keep an eye on your symptoms. If they worsen or persist for more than twenty-four hours, reach out to your PCP. Always contact your healthcare provider if you develop a fever.

7. Avoid Topical Products: Resist the urge to soak your breasts with saline, castor oil, or other topical products. These can interfere with your body's natural adjustment process.[30]

Rule of Thumb: When it comes to treating engorgement, less is more. Stick with gentle approaches like cold therapy and comfortable support rather than aggressive treatments. For a deep dive into the medical aspects, check out Dr. Katrina Mitchell's *Physician Guide to Breastfeeding* in the Resources section.

Finding Your Flow: From Overflow to Just Right

Listen, engorgement is a totally normal part of your breastfeeding journey; it doesn't mean you're doing anything wrong. The good news is it's usually temporary. Most moms find relief within forty-eight to seventy-two hours as their body adjusts and finds its flow. If you experience engorgement that does not begin to improve within seventy-two hours, I advise talking to an IBCLC or breastfeeding and lactation medicine physician (NABBLM-C).[31] Just remember that your body is doing exactly what it's supposed to do—sometimes a little *too* enthusiastically.

And if you're sitting there with ice packs stuffed in your bra right now, wondering if this will ever end—I promise you, it will get better. You're not in this alone, so reach out for support when you need it. That's what lactation consultants like me are here for!

30 ABM Clinical Protocol #36, "Engorgement," Revised 2022.

31 North American Board of Breastfeeding and Lactation Medicine (NABBLM), "Certification," accessed April 5, 2025, https://nabblm.org/certification/.

Mom-to-Mom Insight: "I wish I was better educated on engorgement before leaving the hospital. The pain and engorgement during the first week can be so severe that it can be discouraging. I wish I knew [then] it was only temporary."
—Lactation Consultant at Milk Diva Isabel Price

CHAPTER 9:

IF LATCHING GETS DIFFICULT

I wish I'd known...

A rocky start with latching doesn't mean the end of breastfeeding. There are more ways to feed your baby than social media shows you, and using them while seeking help toward getting back to breastfeeding doesn't make you any less of a breastfeeding mama.

During your baby's first week of life, latching issues can throw a wrench in your breastfeeding plans. Trust me, I've been there—staring down at my baby, wondering why something so "natural" suddenly feels like we're speaking different languages. Take a deep breath, mama. There are plenty of approaches you can try if these situations pop up. Think of these methods as your temporary tool kit until you can connect with a qualified lactation consultant (which, remember from the beginning of this book, should be a top priority!). Just a heads-up, though—don't DIY these solutions for more than a week without professional eyes on the situation. Band-Aid fixes can sometimes create bigger problems down the road if they're not properly evaluated.

Breast Alternatives When Your Baby Can't Latch

First, becoming proficient at hand expression can be a game changer during your baby's initial days. (Again, check out the guide in the Resources section—it's worth bookmarking!) This skill allows you to gently and efficiently remove milk from your breasts using your hands and then offer it to your baby. It ensures that your baby receives the nourishment they need, even when latching difficulties arise (like when your baby struggles to stay awake at the breast).

Once you've expressed some of that liquid gold, you're probably wondering, *Now what? How do I get this milk into my baby without using a bottle?* Let's talk about some alternatives that won't interfere with breastfeeding.

Spoon-Feeding and Cup Feeding

Spoon-feeding and cup feeding are gentle and effective ways to offer your milk to your baby without the use of a bottle. Spoon-feeding involves placing a small amount of milk on a spoon and gently allowing your baby to sip it, while cup feeding involves using a soft-sided cup to tip milk to your baby's lips for them to sip. Just make sure to have a bib or an absorbent cloth ready; your baby might get a bit messy.

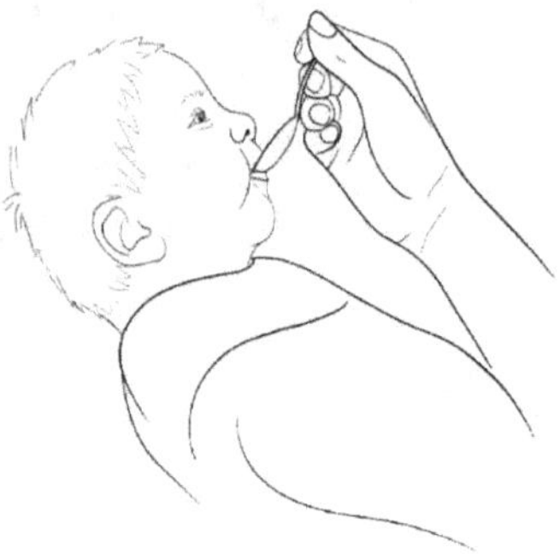

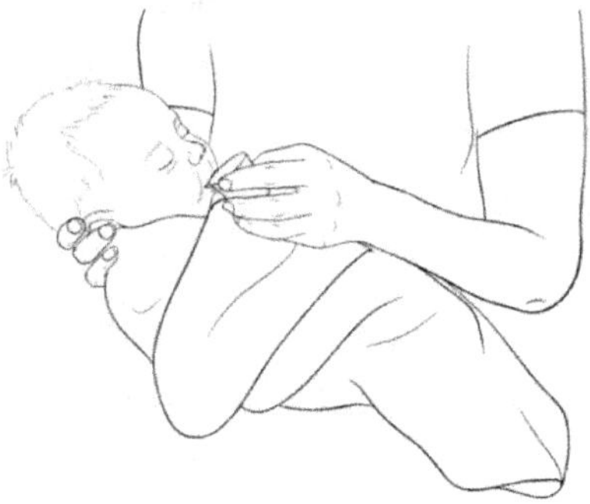

Syringe Feeding

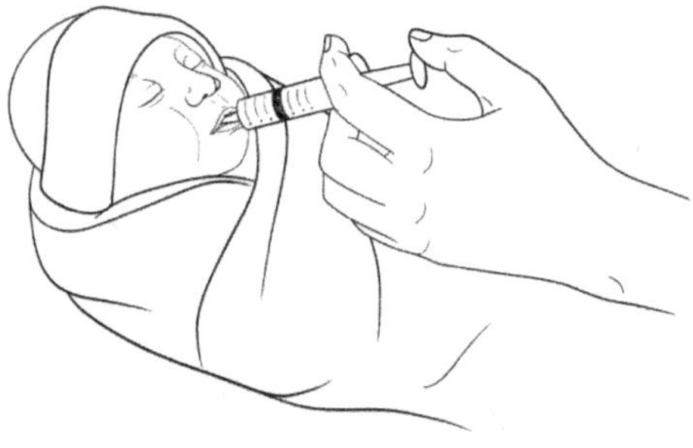

For babies who struggle with latching, a needleless feeding syringe can be a useful tool. After you've hand expressed your milk into a small medicine cup or similar container, you'll suck the milk up into the syringe by pulling back on the plunger while the tip is in the milk). Syringe feeding involves delivering this milk drop by drop to your baby. If your baby can latch but requires additional support, gently introduce the syringe, filled with expressed breast milk, at the corner of your baby's mouth. Make sure to pay close attention to their cues. Go at your baby's pace. Watch for swallowing, pauses in breathing, or turning away, which are your baby's ways of saying

"Slow down" or "I need a break," because even with a syringe, we want to follow the baby's lead, not push an agenda.

Finger Feeding

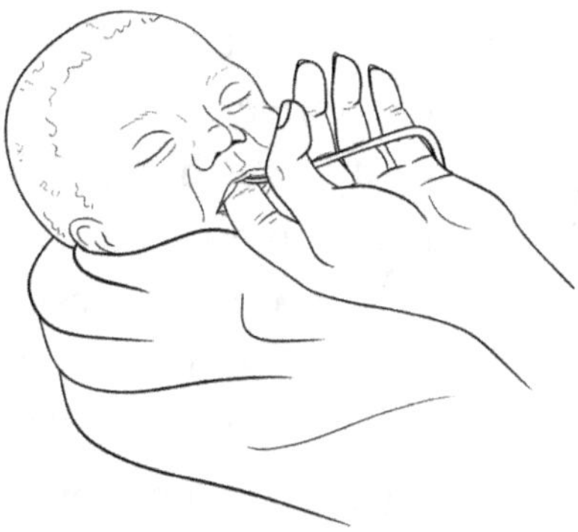

Finger feeding is a technique designed for babies who haven't latched yet or are dealing with latching difficulties. With this method, you use what's called a supplemental nursing system (SNS)—a special thin pediatric feeding tube attached to your clean finger. You can often get this tubing from your hospital before discharge—just ask your nurse or lactation consultant. If they don't provide it, you'll need to purchase an SNS online or through a medical supply company.

Once you have your supplies ready, here's what you do: Gently tickle your baby's lips with your finger, allowing them to latch onto your finger with the feeding tube attached. Your baby can then draw fluid through the tubing, helping them develop proper sucking techniques. Always ensure your hands are thoroughly washed with soap and water prior to finger feeding, and consider using a disposable glove.

At-Breast Supplementer

An at-breast supplementer also uses the thin pediatric feeding tube to bring milk from a device like a bottle all the way to your nipple. Your baby latches to the breast and pulls milk from both the tube and your breast simultaneously. It's particularly beneficial if you're concerned about low milk supply because these devices stimulate the nerves in your breast, encouraging more milk

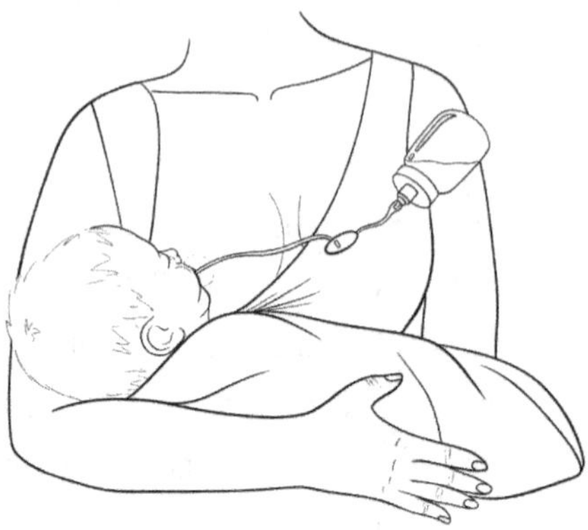

production while providing the required supplement.

While this system sounds like a fantastic solution, I need to be honest with you—it's much more cumbersome and tricky to use than it sounds. You have to position the tube just right at the correct part of your nipple, tape it securely, and then hope your baby's hands don't accidentally pull the whole thing out during feeding. Though you might find instructional videos online (and you can even create a homemade version following instructions from experts like Dr. Jack Newman), this is definitely a tool best used with guidance from a lactation consultant or nurse who can help you avoid the frustration of multiple failed attempts.

Paced Bottle-Feeding

Paced bottle-feeding, which we first mentioned in chapter 4, is a method that mimics breastfeeding to help prevent nipple or flow preference. Hold your baby in an upright position, feed them with a bottle with a slow-flow nipple, and offer breaks just as you would at the breast. It should take your baby about fifteen minutes to drink a bottle. If they are chugging their bottle in five minutes, there is a high likelihood they will start preferring the flow of the bottle over the breast. This approach helps your baby switch between breast and bottle with ease.

Note that bottle refusal is an extremely difficult obstacle to overcome. If you plan to use a bottle in the future, you should definitely seek the counsel of an experienced lactation consultant between three to six weeks of life to introduce a bottle in a manner that complements and protects breastfeeding. This can help prevent your baby from refusing the bottle as they get older. Of course, this step is only necessary if you plan to offer your baby a bottle (e.g., if you're traveling for work, going away for a weekend, or having a planned surgery). For more details on bottle selection, paced bottle-feeding, and nipple shape styles, refer back to chapter 4 and check out the Resources section.

> **Rule of Thumb:** If for any reason you start using a nipple shield, immediately seek the support of a lactation consultant to quickly wean off of the nipple shield, because long-term nipple shield use can lead to low milk supply and low milk transfer to the baby.[32]

Finding Your Flow: When *Plan* A Meets Reality

Navigating breastfeeding challenges requires a balanced approach—you need immediate solutions while working toward long-term success. While I've given you several options like spoon-feeding, cup feeding, syringe feeding, finger feeding, and at-breast supplementation, I want to be crystal clear: you don't need to become an expert at all of these techniques!

Pick *one* method that seems most doable for your situation and get proper guidance on it. The hospital is the perfect place to learn these techniques; ask your nurse or lactation consultant to demonstrate your chosen method before you go home. Most of these alternatives (except for paced bottle-feeding, which is fairly straightforward) should be practiced with professional guidance first. Trying to master multiple feeding methods simultaneously is a recipe for frustration and overwhelm.

32 Frontiers in Public Health, "The Use of Nipple Shields: A Review," November 1, 2016.

These alternative feeding methods are temporary solutions to ensure your baby gets the calories they need while you address the root causes of latching difficulties. Seeking help from an IBCLC is crucial for long-term success. They can monitor your baby's health and weight gain while helping you work toward more comfortable and effective breastfeeding.

Remember, despite initial challenges, professional support ensures you're not navigating this journey alone—and with the right guidance, most latching issues can be resolved, allowing you to find your unique breastfeeding flow.

Mom-to-Mom Insight: "Ask for help! I wish I'd known how quickly a bad latch in those first days can cause excruciating pain that can then take a long while to heal. I had a hospital birth, and I wish I'd asked the nurses for help with every latch in the very beginning rather than worrying that I was bothering them or feeling like I should know after just a couple of sessions with help. With my second, in spite of previous experience, I asked for help checking the latch every time in those first few days without shame, and my journey was off to a much better start because of it." —former patient S.H.

CHAPTER 10:

THE STRAIGHT TALK ON TONGUE-TIES

I wish I'd known...

"They can stick their tongue out, so no tongue-tie" is like saying "The car moves forward, so the brakes must work." Finding the right provider who actually knows how to perform a full functional *and* structural assessment can save you months of struggling and second-guessing.

Tongue-ties are a very controversial issue, and this book is not intended to be an exhaustive manual or step-by-step guide to identifying and overcoming feeding issues related to tongue-ties. However, I would like to share my qualifications and experience with helping families overcome feeding problems related to tongue-ties. Then, I'll share a few tips to consider if you think your baby may be suffering from feeding issues related to a tongue-tie.

When I first began my journey as a lactation consultant, I'll admit I was skeptical about tongue-ties. *Another fad diagnosis*, I thought. Now, after years of clinical experience and seeing both the overdiagnosis *and* the missed cases, I've landed firmly in the middle ground. I've witnessed the heartbreak of mothers who bounced from provider to provider, each giving conflicting opinions. I've also seen the families who had unnecessary procedures that didn't solve their feeding issues. But perhaps most memorable was the nine-month-old patient who came to me struggling with solid foods—aspirating (which means that milk, formula, or food accidentally goes into their airway, aka windpipe, instead of their stomach), requiring weekly speech and occupational therapy and swallow studies—all because a tongue-tie wasn't identified and addressed earlier. These types of experiences shaped my nuanced approach to tongue-ties that I'm sharing with you now.

What Do I Know About Tongue-Ties?

I'm deeply passionate about making your breastfeeding journey as smooth and successful as possible. Over the years, I've worked extensively with infants experiencing feeding challenges due to oral dysfunction, including those related to tongue-tie. I'm proud to be part of a highly respected pediatric dental clinic led by Dr. Poplin, where I'm part of a team that performs comprehensive functional and structural assessments on babies to determine if there is a tongue-tie or other oral restriction present. In this collaborative care setting, Dr. Poplin and I have been able to learn from each other's expertise—combining his dental knowledge with my lactation experience—allowing us to provide the most accurate assessments and recommendations for each family. Together, we evaluate and assess hundreds of infants each year, developing comprehensive treatment plans tailored to each family's specific goals. My role often involves working closely with families to explore nonsurgical interventions before considering a frenectomy or frenotomy (fancy terms for a tongue-tie release procedure).

One of the aspects I'm particularly proud of is our clinic's approach to tongue-tie management. We emphasize reducing the need for surgical procedures whenever possible, opting instead for nonsurgical interventions like expert lactation support and pediatric manual therapy. This philosophy is not only more conservative but also incredibly effective. I've shared these evidence-based approaches in various publications, including articles in parenting magazines. In fact, our clinic's frenectomy rate is about 53%, which means nearly half of the patients referred to us never require a procedure. By providing thorough evaluations and targeted interventions, we've been able to help countless babies resolve their feeding issues without the need for surgical procedures. Our work at the clinic has transformed it into what many now recognize as a Center of Excellence for treating infants with tongue-tie.

This distinction is largely thanks to the collaborative approach we take, which was initially inspired by the innovative work of Autumn Henning, CCC-SLP, COM, IBCLC. Her insights into tongue-tie management helped shape our model of care, emphasizing the importance of collaboration and incorporating noninvasive treatment methods before considering a surgical procedure.

Beyond my clinical work, I have had the opportunity to share our successes and best practices at national medical conferences, contributing to the broader conversation around the management of babies with tongue-tie. So, when it comes to addressing tongue-ties and enhancing feeding experiences for both infants and their families, I bring a wealth of experience and expertise. My ultimate goal is to support you on your unique breastfeeding journey, offering the guidance and assistance you need to thrive. As we continue, I'll share some key tips and insights I've gathered in my years as an IBCLC to help you navigate your journey with tongue-tie.

After sharing all my expertise, I feel I should also share a concern. Tongue-tie diagnosis has become something of a trend in some circles. There are providers out there who may be making recommendations with their wallet in mind rather than your baby's best interests. That's why finding the right help is so crucial.

What Should You Do If You Think Your Baby Has a Tongue-Tie?

If you're concerned that your baby might have a tongue-tie, it's important to get the right kind of help. Tongue-tie is a condition that can affect breastfeeding, and having accurate information and guidance can make a big difference in your breastfeeding journey.

Here's a simple breakdown of what you should do:

Start by Consulting a Qualified Lactation Consultant

Just like you'd want a specialized contractor to build a house in an earthquake-prone area, you want a lactation consultant who specializes in managing tongue-ties to guide you. Finding the right expert can seem overwhelming, but I'm here to make it easier.

Use Professional Directories

You can also look for lactation consultants through professional directories like the International Affiliation of Tongue-Tie Professionals (IATP) or the International Consortium of Oral Ankylofrenula Professionals (ICAP). These directories can help you find someone who is well-trained in dealing with tongue-ties.

Ask the Right Questions

When you talk to a potential lactation consultant, ask about their experience and approach. Here are a few questions that can help:

- How many clients have you helped with tongue-tie issues, and what percentage of them were able to reach their breastfeeding goals? (They may not have an exact percentage, but they should be able to tell you if they've helped the majority of their patients, about half, or just a quarter. Look for someone who has successfully helped more than 60–70 percent of their tongue-tie patients reach their breastfeeding goals.)

- How many lactation consultations do you typically conduct each month? (Look for someone who handles at least thirty or more, as this suggests a high level of experience.)

- What kind of hands-on training have you received in assessing and managing tongue-ties? (Please understand that a five-to-eight-hour online course cannot take the place of real, hands-on training with an experienced mentor.)

- How important is manual therapy (aka body work) in the plan of care when addressing tongue-ties? (If the provider says it's not usually necessary, then please continue your search. Clearly they do not have a full understanding of anatomy and physiology of the tongue and infant feeding.)

- How do you approach care when there are different opinions on treatment options? (This will help you gauge whether the consultant will be open-minded and supportive rather than pressuring or guilting you into following a specific course of action.)

Join a Support Group

Consider joining a local or online tongue-tie support group. These groups are filled with parents who have been in your shoes and can often recommend lactation consultants who helped them successfully manage tongue-tie issues. Word-of-mouth recommendations from parents who have been through similar experiences can be incredibly valuable.

Check Their Online Presence

Look at the consultant's website and social media. If they have specialized training in dealing with tongue-ties, they will often highlight this prominently. On the other hand, if they don't have much experience or confidence in this area, it may not be mentioned as much or at all. Also, pay attention to the tone and values conveyed in their online content to see if they align with your needs and preferences. By following these steps and asking the right questions, you'll be well on your way to finding the right support for managing your baby's tongue-tie and ensuring a smoother breastfeeding experience. Remember, the right lactation consultant will be someone who listens to your concerns, respects your choices, and provides the guidance you need without judgment or pressure.

Avoid Hasty Decisions

I know what you might be thinking: *But my baby is struggling* now! I hear you, mama. That protective instinct to fix things immediately is powerful. But here's what I've learned from thousands of cases: releasing a tongue-tie is *not* a magic fix. Anyone who promises you instant breastfeeding bliss after a quick snip is selling you a fantasy, not reality.

Rushing the process of addressing a tongue-tie could potentially exacerbate your issues or lead to further complications. A tongue-tie release procedure, in isolation, isn't a guaranteed path to long-term breastfeeding success. Genuine success requires a thoughtful, strategic, team-based approach involving the family, a lactation consultant, potentially a manual therapist (like a pediatric chiropractor or physical therapist), and, ultimately, an experienced tongue-tie release provider, who is often a specially trained pediatric dentist.

However, there's a crucial aspect to keep in mind: your attitude plays a significant role in achieving your feeding goals. If you rush the process, skip essential steps, or attempt shortcuts, you could find yourself grappling with issues for far longer than if you had followed the expert guidance provided by your lactation consultant. Patience, dedication, and a systematic approach are your allies in this journey. I completely understand that the urge to rush might stem from deep concern for your baby, especially when you're worried about them not getting enough to eat. Know that this is a natural response rooted in your love and desire to provide for your child. But it's important to remember that taking the time to follow a well-rounded, expert-guided approach will ultimately give you the best chance at long-term success in your baby getting the nourishment they need.

The Real Impact of Tongue-Ties

Throughout my years hosting The Boob Business Podcast and in my clinical practice, I've identified tongue-ties as one of the major roadblocks that can completely derail a new mom's breastfeeding journey. It's often the challenge they couldn't recover from with their first baby and why they're seeking a fresh start with their second.

My goal is not to scare anyone into having a tongue-tie release procedure, but I think it's important to know some of the complications that have been linked to unresolved ties. Beyond the immediate breastfeeding challenges, untreated tongue-ties can lead to difficulty with solid foods, including choking and swallowing difficulties. Children may experience challenges with speech development; sleep issues, including sleep apnea; and airway problems that can continue into adulthood. Many also develop generalized head and neck tension that can cause discomfort for years to come.[33]

What breaks my heart is seeing these downstream effects when ties aren't addressed early. Remember that nine-month-old patient I mentioned? By the time that family found us, they were deep into weekly therapy appointments and medical procedures—all potentially preventable with early identification and proper treatment.

At the same time, I've witnessed the disappointment when a tongue-tie release doesn't instantly solve feeding problems as promised. This is why I take such a team-based approach—the procedure itself is just one piece of a complex puzzle that includes proper assessment, supportive therapies, and realistic expectations.

---

33 Silicon Valley Pediatric Dentistry, "Can a Child Eat Solid Food with a Lip or Tongue Tie?" March 17, 2025.

For the record, I don't believe every baby with a suspected tongue-tie needs a release procedure. It's genuinely one of the most nuanced issues in infant feeding, which is exactly why finding experienced providers who can give you honest, personalized guidance (not just a quick diagnosis and referral) is absolutely critical.

Choosing the Right Person to Check for Tongue-Tie

Identifying and treating a tongue-tie properly requires a team approach, similar to how orthopedic issues are handled. Just as a knee problem requires both functional and structural assessment before deciding on physical therapy or surgery, tongue-ties need a comprehensive evaluation process.

First, you'll need a functional assessment from a specially trained pediatrician, lactation consultant, speech language pathologist, or feeding therapist. These professionals evaluate if your baby's tongue can move appropriately and identify any oral motor-skill deficits. Based on their findings, they'll recommend appropriate next steps, which often include oral therapy and exercises. If the deficits are significant, they'll likely recommend therapeutic exercises while also referring you to a specially trained doctor for another structural assessment.

During this second structural assessment is when your baby typically receives an official diagnosis of ankyloglossia (the medical term for tongue-tie), if one is present. If your baby is diagnosed with a tongue-tie and a procedure is recommended, the provider should teach you how to perform the post-procedure care. This is crucial—you should actually put gloves on and practice the post-procedure stretches on your baby *before* making your final decision.

I recommend taking a few days to practice these stretches at home before returning for the procedure. This preparation helps both you and your baby know what to expect, improving your baby's acceptance and your confidence in performing the necessary aftercare.

After a procedure is performed, you should have a post-procedure checkup with the doctor who performed it within three to seven days, as well as a follow-up appointment with your lactation consultant or feeding therapist to ensure breastfeeding is improving.

Finding Your Flow: Separating Fact from Fiction

Here's a dangerous myth I need to bust: babies do not "grow out of" a tongue-tie, and it's highly unlikely that a tie will randomly tear on its own. I've heard these misconceptions repeated by well-meaning providers who simply don't have specialized training in this area. These myths can lead families to delay proper evaluation and treatment, often resulting in prolonged feeding difficulties.

It is essential to take time and care with this evaluation process to make sure your baby gets the right diagnosis and care they need. So don't be afraid to ask questions and seek someone who knows their stuff when it comes to tongue-ties.

> **Mom-to-Mom Insight:** "Tongue-ties can be a significant impediment to a breastfeeding journey, and many practitioners (particularly pediatricians) are not trained in identifying them. If you suspect your child may be tongue-tied, make sure you find an experienced IBCLC who can properly diagnose it and help you find the proper treatment, as well as educate you on the process for before and after the procedure."
> —former patient Reann Kobitz

CHAPTER 11:

SUPPLEMENTING SMARTS AND MILK STORAGE SECRETS

I wish I'd known...

Supplementing and milk storage decisions should be based on what your baby needs right now, not on creating a massive freezer stash for the future. Also, don't be too overzealous about freezing a bunch of milk before you test to see if it changes flavor after being frozen; otherwise this could lead to having a freezer full of milk your baby won't accept.

Human milk was designed to meet all a baby's intricate nutritional needs, but sometimes human milk is not an option for some families. In these cases, the next closest substitute is using donor breast milk, especially for preterm babies. When donor milk is not available, then infant formula is the next best alternative. The world of supplementation can be a bit overwhelming, and often, you'll hear differing opinions from various sources. So let's break down the essentials and help you make an informed choice for your little one.

First, it's crucial to understand why some providers may recommend supplementing, even for breastfeeding moms. In certain situations, like for first-time mothers, those who had a cesarean section, or women with preeclampsia, it may take more than five to seven days before breast milk production aligns with a baby's metabolic needs.[34] In such cases, immediate action is necessary to ensure your baby is nourished while you're working toward an increased milk supply. In addition, babies who are experiencing jaundice and who have high levels of bilirubin may become too sleepy to breastfeed effectively. In this situation, supplementation may be crucial to the newborn's ability to thrive.

Exploring Your Supplementation Options: Donor Breast Milk and Formula

Supplementation in the context of feeding a baby refers to providing additional nutrition beyond what the baby is receiving from breastfeeding alone. This can be necessary in situations where the baby is not gaining enough weight, has specific nutritional needs, or when breastfeeding alone is not meeting the baby's nutritional requirements.

34 PubMed Central, "The Impact of Caesarean Section on Breastfeeding Initiation and Duration," April 26, 2016.

Supplementation can take various forms:

1. **Expressed Breast Milk:** Feeding the baby with pumped breast milk either through a bottle or another feeding method to supplement breastfeeding

2. **Donor Milk:** Breast milk provided by screened donors to supplement a baby's nutrition, ensuring they receive the benefits of human milk when the mother's own milk is unavailable or insufficient

3. **Formula Supplementation:** Giving the baby infant formula alongside breastfeeding to ensure they receive enough nutrients and calories

If you need to supplement, your own expressed milk is almost always the best first choice—you can offer it to your baby using any of those feeding methods we talked about in chapter 9.

The next best option when supplementing is donor breast milk, when available. Breast milk is designed to be the easiest and most nutrient-dense form of nourishment for your baby. Donor breast milk from a milk bank undergoes a pasteurization process and is generally considered very safe. However, it's worth noting that access to donor breast milk can be limited and may involve risks if it's not from a regulated milk bank.

If donor breast milk isn't an option for you, the next best choice is ready-to-feed formula. Newborns less than two months old, those who are premature, or those with weakened immune systems should receive sterile formula.[35] Liquid formula is sterile and considered the safest option.

35 Centers for Disease Control and Prevention (CDC), "Prepare and Store Powdered Infant For-

Please be sure to understand the risks associated with each of the supplementation options, including the risks of formula use. To protect your breastfeeding relationship when supplementing, continue latching your baby to your breast frequently or use a breast pump at least eight times in twenty-four hours.

Okay, let's talk formula basics. I'm going to cut through the marketing noise and give you the straight talk about what really matters.

Demystifying Formula Choices

Let me set your mind at ease about formula options. All infant formulas sold in the United States are regulated by the FDA,[36] which requires manufacturers to register and meet specific nutritional and safety standards. What does this mean for you? It means that generic formulas aren't inherently inferior to the fancy branded ones with the cute commercials. In fact, their nutritional compositions are remarkably similar! So if you're supplementing and watching your budget (and who isn't these days?), know that you can choose a more affordable option without shortchanging your baby on nutrition. The expensive marketing doesn't always translate to a superior product when it comes to formula.

Here are key aspects to consider:

1. Protein Source: You'll find cow's milk protein and soy protein among the most common options. For cow's milk protein, it's further broken down into casein and whey. The key here is to know that casein is more difficult for your baby to digest than

---

mula in an Emergency," May 6, 2024.

36 U.S. Food and Drug Administration, "Infant Formula," last modified January 10, 2025, accessed April 5, 2025, https://www.fda.gov/food/resources-you-food/infant-formula.

whey.[37] So, when selecting an infant formula for your newborn, a whey-based formula may be a better option for your newborn.

Another aspect to consider is the size of the cow's milk protein molecule. This is especially important during the first few months, when your newborn's digestive system is still developing. During this time, you should consider selecting a formula with partially hydrolyzed protein, which is easier to digest.[38]

2. Carbohydrate Source: Lactose is the carbohydrate found in breast milk and is the ideal carbohydrate source when choosing a formula. It's important to know that more than 99 percent of all babies have the enzymes necessary to digest lactose. True lactose intolerance generally appears after puberty,[39] so your baby may not be lactose intolerant even if you are.

3. Fat Source: This could be palm olein oil or coconut oil. Opt for formulas with coconut oil listed before palm oil, or even better, those with 100 percent coconut oil. Coconut oil may be gentler on the digestive system and aid in better nutrient absorption in addition to reducing the risk of chronic constipation. Palm oil is fine for healthy term babies but not recommended for preterm infants, as it may affect bone density.[40]

Formula Shopping Tips

When choosing a formula, don't be swayed by flashy packaging or marketing terms such as "comfort proteins," "easy digestion,"

---

37 PubMed Central, "Adjustment of Whey:Casein Ratio from 20:80 to 60:40 in Milk Formulations," March 19, 2021.

38 PubMed Central, "A Partially Hydrolyzed Whey Infant Formula Supports Appropriate Growth in Healthy Term Infants," October 6, 2020.

39 Medscape, "Pediatric Lactose Intolerance: Background, Pathophysiology, Etiology," December 3, 2024.

40 PubMed Central, "Reduced Bone Mineralization in Infants Fed Palm Olein-Containing Formula," May 22, 2003.

"immune support," or "brain building." (Seriously, the marketing departments deserve gold stars for creativity, but we're looking for substance here!) The claims on formula packaging can be as misleading as the "made with real fruit!" assertions on sugary children's cereals.

While formula ingredients are regulated, the marketing claims on the front of packages often create impressions that don't tell the whole story. For example, when a formula advertises "added DHA for brain development," they've included a minimal amount of this nutrient—not necessarily enough to have the suggested impact. Or when they claim to contain "human milk oligosaccharides (HMOs) just like breast milk," they typically include just two types, while breast milk naturally contains well over 100 different varieties.

Rule of Thumb: The fancier the formula label and the more promises it makes, the more you're likely paying for marketing, not better nutrition. U.S. formulas must meet the same nutritional standards. The only real differences are in things like molecule structure and pre-/probiotics, not in how well they'll nourish your baby.

Instead, head straight to the ingredient list. Focus on the protein, carbohydrate, and fat sources that suit your baby's needs. For newborns under three months of age, a good choice is partially hydrolyzed cow's milk and whey for protein, lactose for carbohydrates, and coconut oil for fat.[41] Of course if your baby has been prescribed or recommended to have a special type of formula due to prematurity, allergies or digestive issues, please always follow your doctor's advice.

41 PubMed Central (PMC), "Partial Hydrolyzed Protein as a Protein Source for Infant Feeding," April 21, 2022.

Insider Secret: I know it can be difficult to find an organic and grass-fed infant formula that meets the suggested requirements above, but please understand that an organic, grass-fed formula that is made from a whole cow's milk protein (compared to a partially hydrolyzed cow's milk protein) won't make it easier for your baby to digest during these delicate first few weeks of life.

For further guidance on formula selection, I recommend checking out Dr. Bridget Young's website, Baby Formula Expert, which has been featured in several national publications, along with my podcast interview of her, which can be found in the Resources section.

Remember that it's crucial to prepare formula safely if you're not using ready-to-feed formula. You can find detailed guidelines on formula preparation from the Centers for Disease Control and Prevention (CDC).[42] It's important to understand why formula might be recommended for certain situations. When selecting a formula, focus on protein, carbohydrate, and fat sources that suit your baby's needs, and choose formulas that closely mimic breast milk composition for the best results. In your journey as a new parent, remember that there is no one-size-fits-all approach. Every baby and every parent is unique. Be open to adjusting your approach as you get to know your baby better, and always seek support and guidance from healthcare professionals when needed.

Infant Formula Preparation and Storage

When it comes to formula feeding, ensuring proper preparation and storage is paramount for your baby's health. Let's look at the

42 Centers for Disease Control and Prevention (CDC), "Infant Formula Preparation and Storage," CDC, April 5, 2025.

guidelines laid out by the World Health Organization (WHO)[43] to provide your little one with the best possible nourishment.

Understanding the Importance of Proper Formula Preparation

1. Hygiene First: Before you even think about preparing the formula, ensure that your hands are thoroughly washed. Sterilize all feeding equipment by boiling it for at least ten minutes.

2. Follow the Mixing Instructions: Different formulas come with different mixing instructions. Pay close attention to the guidelines provided on the formula tin. Getting the right ratio of water to formula is crucial for your baby's health. Be sure to add the water to the container before adding the formula powder. This will help prevent some of the complications that can occur if the solution is too concentrated.[44]

3. Water Quality: If you're using tap water, make sure it's safe to drink. The water does not need to have any added ingredients, such as fluoride or electrolytes. To kill germs like cronobacter that are sometimes found in powdered infant formula, the formula must be mixed with very hot water.[45] Boil the water and then wait about five minutes before mixing with powdered infant formula.

Storage Guidelines for Prepared Formula

1. Refrigeration: Once you've prepared the formula, it needs to be consumed or stored in the refrigerator within two hours. Any formula left in the bottle after a feed should be discarded.

---

43 World Health Organization (WHO), Safe Preparation, Storage and Handling of Powdered Infant Formula: Guidelines, WHO, 2007.

44 PubMed Central, "Hypernatremic Dehydration Due to Concentrated Infant Formula," May 22, 2009.

45 Centers for Disease Control and Prevention (CDC), "Infant Formula Preparation and Storage," December 19, 2024.

2. Short Shelf Life: Prepared formula has a short shelf life. If stored in a refrigerator, use it within twenty-four hours. If it's been at room temperature for more than two hours, discard it.

3. Do Not Freeze: Unlike breast milk, formula should not be frozen. Freezing alters its consistency and can affect its nutritional value.[46]

If you're using formula, I recommend following the World Health Organization's guidelines for safe preparation and storage.[47] These evidence-based practices are crucial for reducing infection risk and protecting your baby's health. Now, let's shift gears and talk about breast milk storage. Trust me, future you will thank present you for mastering these basics now.

Breast Milk Storage and Preparation

Breast milk storage is a crucial aspect of your breastfeeding journey. Proper storage ensures that your breast milk remains a safe form of nutrition for your baby. Let's explore the intricacies of refrigeration, freezing, and daily breast milk expression.

Refrigeration: Safeguarding Freshness

1. Container Choice: Use clean, glass or BPA-free plastic containers with secure lids for your breast milk.

2. Proper Hygiene: Wash your hands before handling breast milk, and ensure all surfaces and containers are clean.

46 PubMed Central, "Effect of Freezing Time on Macronutrients and Energy Content of Human Milk," January 1, 2012.

47 World Health Organization, Safe Preparation, Storage and Handling of Powdered Infant Formula: Guidelines, Geneva: WHO, 2007. ISBN: 9789241595414. Accessed April 8, 2025. https://www.who.int/publications/i/item/9789241595414.

3. Time and Date Stamp: Label each container with the date of expression. This practice helps you prioritize using breast milk in the order it was produced, ensuring optimal freshness.

4. Prompt Refrigeration: Refrigerate your expressed milk quickly, aiming to always keep it at a temperature range of 32–39°F (0–4°C).[48]

5. Strategic Placement: Store breast milk toward the back of the fridge for consistent temperatures, avoiding the warmer areas near the door.

6. Chilling Duration: Freshly expressed milk stays fresh in the fridge for four to eight days.[49] Be sure to smell and taste the breast milk before offering it to your baby to ensure it has not spoiled.

Freezing Wisdom: Planning for the Future

1. Portion Control: Freeze breast milk in small portions. I suggest 2–4 ounces (about 60–120 milliliters) for efficient thawing and minimal waste.

2. Freezer-Ready Containers: Invest in airtight, freezer-friendly bags or containers. Ensure they can withstand freezing temperatures and will not crack or leak.

3. Expansion Consideration: Allow space at the top of your container or bag for liquid expansion during freezing.

4. Freezer Setting: Maintain your freezer at 0°F (-18°C) or below to retain nutrient quality.[50]

---

48 Academy of Breastfeeding Medicine (ABM), Clinical Protocol #8: Human Milk Storage Information for Home Use for Full-Term Infants, Revised 2017.

49 PubMed Central, "Saving Expressed Breast Milk," December 6, 2003.

50 Helmer Scientific, "Safely Storing Breast Milk in the Refrigerator," March 2022.

5. Thawing Gradually: Plan ahead for thawing by moving frozen breast milk to the fridge the night before. Avoid microwaving the breast milk, as this could damage the nutrients.[51]

6. Thawing Quickly: For rapid thawing, place the sealed container or bag under cool running water or in a bowl of warm water.

Insider Secret: Did you know that your breastmilk's flavor may taste differently after being frozen, and your baby may not drink it? This is caused by a naturally occurring enzyme in human milk called lipase. Some women have higher levels of lipase in their milk which can change the taste and smell of the milk after being frozen. To prevent having a freezer stash full of milk your baby won't drink because it tastes different, I recommend smelling and tasting a fresh sample of your milk, then freezing it. After thawing, smell and taste it again. Watch for any foul odor or taste, or the development of soapy or metallic taste or smell. If there is no significant change, then go ahead and freeze your milk. If the taste or smell changes significantly or becomes unpleasant, you likely have high lipase milk and will need to explore other options before building your freezer stash.

Pumping Wisdom: Quality Over Quantity

Pumping isn't about filling your freezer to the brim. Sometimes pumping is not even necessary; however, if you plan to work outside the home or be away from your baby for a day or two, pumping can be a great way to ensure your baby continues to consume your milk. Instead of focusing on having a freezer full of frozen breast milk, focus on a gradual approach. Store one feed per day (3–4 ounces) for approximately four weeks before your return to work.

51 Mayo Clinic, "Breast Milk Storage: Do's and Don'ts," March 27, 2025

This usually works best if you pump and store your breast milk right after your first morning breastfeeding session. This strategy typically provides an ample supply of stored milk.

Room Temperature Wisdom: Navigating Time Frames
Understanding the dynamics of room temperature storage is crucial for maintaining breast milk quality. Consider these guidelines:

1. **Short Stints:** Freshly expressed milk is safe at room temperature for approximately four to six hours.[52] This flexibility is particularly handy for moments when immediate refrigeration isn't feasible. Picture this—you pump overnight and, instead of navigating the stairs to reach the fridge, you opt for temporary room-temperature storage. It's a practical solution, given the limited time frame and your exhaustion. (Please remember this is *not* true of infant formula. Infant formula *cannot* stay out at room temperature.)

2. **Time Sensitivity:** Any breast milk that has not been consumed within one hour of touching your baby's mouth must be discarded.[53] This protects your baby's health by preventing any potential bacterial growth. By mastering the art of breast milk storage, you're ensuring that every precious drop you produce contributes to your baby's growth and nourishment. Happy expressing and storing!

Finding Your Flow: Feeding with Confidence

Remember when I said preparation is everything? This is exactly what I meant. Whether you're supplementing with formula or storing your liquid gold for future feeds, having this knowledge in your back pocket means one less thing to google in the middle of the night. You don't need to memorize every detail—that's why this book exists

52 HealthyChildren.org, "Storing and Preparing Expressed Breast Milk," March 20, 2024.
53 HealthyChildren.org, "How Long Can Baby Bottles Sit at Room Temperature?" August 5, 2022.

as your trusted guide. What matters is that you now understand the options available and the basics of keeping your baby's nutrition safe and effective, whatever feeding path you find yourself on. And if you're ever unsure? Trust your instincts and reach out to your healthcare provider. You're doing an amazing job navigating these early weeks, mama, and each feeding—whether from breast, bottle, or both—is an act of love. That's what truly matters.

Mom-to-Mom Insight: "If you're struggling, formula exists for a reason. Don't push something if it's causing you more anxiety and stress than you can handle."
—former patient M.B.

PART III:

WHAT I WISH I'D KNOWN IN THE FIRST WEEKS

CHAPTER 12:

HOME SWEET HOME WITH ZERO SLEEP

I wish I'd known...

I was trying to get my baby to sleep through the night starting at three months old because I thought that was the goal. Instead, I wish I would have known what the more realistic, healthy, and attainable sleep patterns actually look like for babies.

You've made it home from the hospital with your tiny human, and somewhere between unpacking those cute little onesies and figuring out how to fold that complicated stroller, it hits you: "Wait... now what?!" Don't worry; I've been exactly where you are—staring at my baby, wondering if life would ever feel normal again.

Those first weeks at home are a beautiful mess of tender moments, overwhelming love, and—let's be real—some serious sleep deprivation. During my first week home with my son, I remember crying over spilled breast milk in the middle of the night while my baby was screaming and my husband was snoring. (Not his fault, but at that moment... it definitely *felt* like his fault.)

Here's what I wish someone had told me then: you don't have to be a sleep-deprived zombie to be a good parent. In fact, getting some solid sleep will make you a better, more patient parent who can actually enjoy those newborn snuggles instead of just surviving them.

In this chapter, we're going to talk straight about sleep and nighttime feeding—the good, the bad, and the bleary-eyed. I'll share some practical strategies that have helped thousands of families in my practice balance the very real needs of a breastfeeding baby with the equally real need for parents to get some rest. Because while those social media posts might show serene mothers peacefully nursing in a perfectly decorated nursery, the reality usually involves spit-up, tears (yours and baby's), and wondering if you'll ever sleep more than two consecutive hours again.

Let's dive in and figure out how to make this work—for your baby, for your milk supply, and most importantly, for your sanity.

The Real Impact of Sleep Deprivation on Breastfeeding

So what actually happens when you're running on fumes? Well, those first few weeks of broken sleep aren't just uncomfortable—they can affect nearly every aspect of your parenting journey. Understanding these effects can help you prioritize rest and recognize when your exhaustion might be influencing how you perceive your breastfeeding success. Trust me, sometimes what feels like a milk supply issue at dawn is actually just your tired brain catastrophizing after the fifth wake-up of the night.

Sleep deprivation is never a fun experience! Here's how it may affect you in the beginning of your baby's life:

Effects on Breastfeeding and Milk Supply

When you're tired, it's easy to question your milk supply and your baby's ability to latch and feed effectively. This anxiety about not producing enough milk can become overwhelming and stressful. The good news is that despite how common sleep deprivation is in the early stages of a baby's life, the overwhelming majority of moms can still produce sufficient milk if they follow effective breastfeeding practices. Your body is remarkably resilient, even when you're exhausted.

Effects on Bonding with and Enjoying Your Newborn

Sleep deprivation can also hinder your ability to bond with your newborn. Those precious moments of gazing into your baby's eyes and relishing their every coo can be marred by exhaustion. The magical moments of connection are often overtaken by the need for sleep.

Effects on Decision-Making

Beyond bonding and milk supply, sleep deprivation can impact your ability to make rational decisions. It's essential to have a clear mind when making choices about your baby's care and feeding, and sleepless nights can cloud your judgment.

When you're severely sleep-deprived, your perspective gets distorted. Small breastfeeding challenges can feel like major crises, and normal baby behaviors might seem like serious problems. For example, maybe the baby is feeding fine but is gassy. When you're exhausted, you may start having thoughts like, *Oh, maybe it's my milk; maybe it's this, maybe it's that*, and you might start to make some irrational or maybe hyperreactive decisions that could interfere with breastfeeding.

Effects on Postpartum Mood

Sleep deprivation is a significant contributor to postpartum mood disorders, such as anxiety and depression. The combination of fragmented sleep and the emotional roller coaster of new motherhood can create a perfect storm for intense mood swings and heightened emotional sensitivity.

When you're severely sleep-deprived, you can find yourself caught in a dangerous cycle—you become irritable and short-tempered, your body releases stress hormones and adrenaline, and then paradoxically, you're too wired to sleep even when given the opportunity. This overstimulation perpetuates anxiety and can significantly worsen your mental health.

If you notice signs of postpartum mood disorders—persistent sadness, excessive worry, difficulty bonding with your baby, or dramatic mood shifts—please contact your healthcare provider right away. These symptoms require professional support and shouldn't be dismissed as normal "baby blues."

Important Safety Information:
If you ever have thoughts of harming yourself or your baby, this is an emergency. The National Maternal Mental Health Hotline provides free, confidential support 24/7 at 1-833-TLC-MAMA (1-833-852-6262). Help is available immediately—you don't need to struggle through these feelings alone.

For more information about recognizing the signs and symptoms of postpartum mood disorders, listen to Episode 23 of The Boob Boss Podcast.[54]

Practical Sleep Setups That Work

Given the overwhelming impact of sleep deprivation, developing a sleep plan is crucial. This plan should aim to provide you with about four hours of uninterrupted sleep overnight. Let me share what I've found works best for the thousands of families I've supported.

The Shift Approach: Your Ticket to Sanity

The best, most practical sleep setup is for each parent to get at least four hours of uninterrupted sleep. This might sound a little controversial, and you're going to hear lots of different advice. But in my experience, that's what works best to help a mom meet her long-term breastfeeding goals, because this is a marathon, not a sprint.

If a mom wakes up every time the baby wants to eat, and if that baby wants to eat every two hours, she's going to quickly start thinking about other ways to survive, including using formula. So instead, I like to have each person (Mom and her support person) take shifts—four-hour shifts.

---

54 https://www.buzzsprout.com/1885195

Here's how it might work: The mom might say, "Okay, I'm going to sleep from 11 P.M. to 3 A.M." So that means Dad or the partner or the nanny or a supportive friend would go into the nursery or the baby's room. Mom pumps at 11 o'clock and leaves milk for her partner to give to the baby at the next feeding. She then puts earphones on or earplugs in, turns on the sound machine, and goes to sleep for four hours.

When Mom wakes up, she tags out with her partner. At that point, she will nurse her baby or pump again, going into the nursery, and her partner will go into the bedroom. They'll get four hours of sleep from, say, 3:30 to 7:30 in the morning.

And then in the morning, they still care for each other, they get along, they're not considering why they did this and why they had this baby, and they're able to make nonemotional, rational decisions.

The Ideal Physical Setup

The most practical sleep setup is to have a separate nursery with a twin-sized bed in the nursery. There's no reason for you to have the nursery in your room where both people sleeping are going to get woken up by every sound the baby makes, because all night long they go, "Uh, uh, uh, uh," making all these sounds.

In this setup, everybody sleeps in their proper place: baby in the crib and the on-duty adult in the twin-size bed. Make sure you have a changing table with a nice dim light—no bright lights because they can bring you and your baby wide awake.

Preparation for Sleep Shifts

Before your sleep shift begins, breastfeed or pump enough to drain your breasts. Set aside the freshly pumped milk so your partner can feed it to your little one during your sleep shift.

Remember, freshly pumped milk is safe at room temperature for four to six hours.

Consider sleeping in a separate room from your baby during your sleep shift so you can enjoy uninterrupted sleep. Listen to white noise sounds or use earplugs to help block out noises. It might take a few nights for you to get used to this separation, but it will help you get deeper, more rejuvenating sleep.

Incorporate your partner or support person in the feeding journey early on. This can help them establish their own rhythm and connection with the baby. It increases their feelings of self-efficacy, reducing any sense of helplessness. Your support person becomes a teammate rather than just a cheerleader. It also makes both of you more understanding and gracious with each other.

What to Expect: Sleep Patterns in the First Month

If you're hoping to understand your newborn's sleep patterns or establish some kind of predictable schedule in those early weeks, I need to be straight with you. Your baby's sleep is going to be a hot mess until about eight weeks. There's no such thing as scheduling. There is no expectation for sleep patterns in these first eight weeks.

Realistic Expectations

Basically, they're waking up every two to three hours at night until somewhere between six and eight weeks of life. I don't generally start seeing babies sleep for longer stretches until around eight weeks, as long as they're being properly fed during the day, meaning getting enough calories. Then you start seeing them stretch out to four-hour stretches overnight.

But at one week, two weeks, four weeks, five weeks? There is no expectation. There should be no scheduling. You should feed that baby on demand.

Why Scheduling Doesn't Work for Newborns

It's crucial to understand that sleep training your baby before three to four months of life is highly discouraged. It is normal for babies to wake up frequently overnight because they cycle in and out of deep sleep quickly.

Frequent nighttime feeds are necessary because your baby's tummy is small relative to their rapid growth. They require small, frequent feedings to maintain steady blood sugar levels and fuel their rapid growth. When your baby seems hungry during the night, it's a genuine need. They are not trying to purposely punish you. Listen to your baby's cues and feed them.

When to Expect Longer Stretches

The journey toward longer sleep stretches is gradual and depends on your baby's growth and feeding patterns. Around six to eight weeks, your baby's stomach capacity increases and their body becomes more efficient at processing breast milk.[55] This physical development, combined with a more mature nervous system, is what typically allows for those first extended sleep periods.

If you want your baby to sleep better at night, focus on making sure they're getting enough calories during their conscious hours. If your baby requires, say, 20 ounces of milk per twenty-four hours at two weeks of age, and you've only fed that baby 12 ounces during the day, giving one large 4-ounce bottle before bed still won't make that big of a difference. The baby needed 20 ounces total, so it's still going to wake up to feed until it gets what it needs.

---

55 La Leche League Canada, "Newborns Have Small Stomachs," January 1, 2022.

Keep in mind this transition doesn't happen overnight (pun intended)—it's a process. You might get one great night with a four-hour stretch followed by a night of frequent wakings. This variation is completely normal as your baby adjusts to their growing body and changing needs.

Signs That Something Might Be Wrong

If the baby is crying and fussing and waking up every hour and a half at night, there is a problem. A baby should be sleeping for two to three hours overnight if we're giving them enough calories during the day.

While you're breastfeeding, you might say, "Well, you don't really know how much milk the baby's getting." But if you work with a lactation consultant, you should be able to know through weighted feeds during your consultation. You're also learning how to tell if the baby is actively swallowing at the breast, and you can know how much time is appropriate.

If your baby is swallowing at the breast for only two minutes on each side and then sleeping the rest of the time, yes, they're going to wake up every hour overnight. But if your baby is nursing, able to stay awake, and swallowing for eight to ten minutes on each side, your baby's getting full feeds—3-4 ounces—and filling up their little milk tank during the day so they're not needing to do that at night.

Nighttime Feeding Realities

One of the great ironies of new motherhood is that you're desperate for sleep, yet your body decides this is the perfect time to ramp up milk production. It feels like your body and baby are conspiring to keep you awake (they're not, of course, but try telling yourself that after the fourth feeding of the night). But there's actually some fascinating biology behind this midnight milk factory, and understanding it can help you work with your body instead of fighting against it.

Biological Importance of Nighttime Milk Production

Here's something fascinating about your body: you'll typically produce the most milk between 2 and 7 A.M. Your prolactin levels (the hormone responsible for milk production) are naturally higher at night due to your circadian rhythm.[56] It's one of nature's curious quirks—you make more milk when you're trying to sleep and less during the day when you're actually up and ready to feed your baby.

Is nighttime feeding especially important for milk supply? Yes, but I'd frame it this way: milk removal at night is particularly valuable for your supply. Think about it—if at 3 P.M. you're only making 2 ounces total, but at 3 A.M. you're making 4 ounces, you want to take advantage of that extra production. Whether your baby is drinking directly or you're pumping to give milk later, make the most of that nighttime abundance, especially if you're working to increase your supply.

And here's something that might make those middle-of-the-night feedings a little more bearable: research shows that breastfeeding moms actually get more sleep overall than formula-feeding moms[57]. I know it doesn't feel like it when you're up for the third time while your partner snores peacefully, but those sleep-promoting hormones released during breastfeeding are working in your favor.

Of course, if you're already producing plenty of milk during the day, you're likely making plenty at night too. In that case, we'd

56 PubMed Central, "Prolactin Circadian Rhythm Persists Throughout Lactation in Women," Neuroendocrinology, January 1990.

57 Therese Doan et al., "Breastfeeding Increases Sleep Duration of New Parents," Journal of Clinical Sleep Medicine 10, no. 3 (2014): 313–319, https://doi.org/10.5664/jcsm.3538.

focus on how to manage that nighttime supply without causing engorgement or mastitis.

In the end, it's these late-night moments when the rest of the world is asleep that form the unbreakable bond between you and your baby. However, your sleep is important as well. Don't hesitate to ask for help from your partner or your support network if these nighttime wakings are causing you mental distress.

Misconception About Formula Helping Babies Sleep Longer
Another misconception is that formula-fed babies sleep longer than breastfed babies. That is not true. What is true, however, is that babies who are well-fed during the day sleep better at night.

Things to Avoid and Recovery Strategies

As much as we focus on what to do during those sleep-deprived early weeks, sometimes knowing what not to do is just as important. When you're running on two hours of sleep and your third cup of coffee, you'll try almost anything that promises relief! Trust me, I get it—if today's world of online shopping had existed when I was breastfeeding (the iPhone wasn't invented then), I would have bought almost anything that promised to help—designer formula, specialty pumps, elaborate bottles, you name it. The desperation for sleep makes even the most budget-conscious parent consider outrageous purchases. Let's talk about some common practices to avoid, along with strategies that will actually help you recover without compromising your breastfeeding journey or your bank account.

Dangerous Practices to Avoid
One of the most dangerous pieces of advice new parents receive is to bundle their babies in layers and keep the room warm. The truth is, overheating is a serious risk for newborns. Your baby

should be wearing just one more layer than what you need to feel comfortable. Skip those thick, fuzzy blankets and keep your home at a reasonable temperature.

I'm also incredibly concerned about devices that are marketed as sleep solutions. These contraptions strap babies down and restrict their natural movement, which might look peaceful but can actually interfere with proper development. Babies need to move their arms and legs! They need to shift positions and wake naturally for feedings.

Many occupational therapists and physical therapists agree: babies shouldn't have their hips and limbs restricted for extended periods.[58] Plus, these deep, uninterrupted sleep periods can cause babies to miss important feedings, which impacts your milk supply. Remember, your baby waking during the night is actually biologically normal and important for their development.

Recovery Strategies That Protect Milk Supply

When you've reached your exhaustion limit—maybe after several nights of waking every ninety minutes—it's time for a recovery strategy. Unfortunately, there's no such thing as truly "catching up" on lost sleep, but you can implement a recovery plan that won't compromise your milk supply.

Here's what works for many families: On a weekend (or whenever your support person is available), say, "I need to get some solid sleep. I'm going to sleep in the guest room and take two four-hour stretches of uninterrupted rest." Before each sleep stretch, pump thoroughly and leave milk for your partner to feed the baby. When

58 Nationwide Children's Hospital, "Exercises: Upper Extremities Infant (Passive)," Reviewed December 2017.

you wake after your first four hours, pump again, then go back for another four-hour sleep cycle.

That eight hours of sleep (broken only by one pumping session) can make you feel like a new person. Your milk supply stays maintained through the pumping, and your mental health gets the reset it desperately needs.

Caffeine and Breast Milk

Good news for you coffee lovers! Caffeine passes into breast milk in such minimal amounts that it rarely affects babies[59]. Despite what you might have heard, having a cup or two of coffee each day is perfectly safe when you're breastfeeding. Breast milk actually contains components that tend to make babies sleepy after feeding well, which counteracts any slight stimulant effect from caffeine. The amount that transfers into your milk is tiny, and the amount that actually becomes bioavailable in your baby's system is even smaller.

The same principle applies to those questions about nighttime milk containing melatonin: while there are small differences in composition between day and night milk, they typically don't make a significant difference in your baby's sleep patterns.

Balancing Bottle-Feeding and Breastfeeding

I've worked with thousands of breastfeeding families, and I've noticed a pattern: parents who allow some strategic bottle-feeding tend to sustain their breastfeeding journey longer than those who refuse all bottles out of fear of "nipple confusion." Here's my take: nipple confusion isn't really about babies being confused—they simply prefer the feeding method that gives them milk with the

59 Shela Akbar Ali Hirani and Allison Ruth Souter, "Effects of Caffeine on Breastfeeding Mothers and Infants: A Scoping Review," Clinical Lactation 15, no. 1 (2024), https://doi.org/10.1891/CL-2023-0036

least effort. This is something we can control through proper bottle-feeding techniques (review chapter 9 for more on pace bottle-feeding).

What's more likely to derail your breastfeeding goals is chronic sleep deprivation. When you're exhausted, every small challenge feels enormous. That slightly gassy baby? Suddenly you're questioning your milk, your diet, your entire approach to feeding. You're more vulnerable to making reactive decisions that can disrupt your breastfeeding relationship.

Using one or two bottles daily (while breastfeeding for the other feeds) gives you breathing room for rest without compromising your breastfeeding relationship. The benefit of that mental clarity and emotional resilience far outweighs the minimal risk of introducing occasional bottles.

Finding Your Flow: One Night at a Time

The first few weeks at home with your baby are a major adjustment—physically, emotionally, and definitely when it comes to your sleep schedule. But here's what I want you to remember: this intense period is temporary. Your baby will eventually sleep longer stretches, you'll develop systems that work for your family, and one day you'll look back on these hazy nights with a mix of wonder and ask, "How did we survive that?!" In the meantime, be gentle with yourself. Some nights your carefully crafted sleep plan will work beautifully. Other nights your baby will have different ideas, and that's okay too. What matters is that you're making intentional choices about how to balance everyone's needs rather than letting exhaustion make those choices for you.

And remember, asking for help isn't just okay—it's essential. Whether it's your partner taking a feeding shift, a friend bringing over a meal, or a lactation consultant helping troubleshoot feeding challenges, support is what will carry you through this time.

You're doing the hard work of nurturing a new human while your body recovers from pregnancy and birth. That deserves grace, rest when you can get it, and maybe a standing ovation. You've got this, one night at a time.

> **Mom-to-Mom Insight:** "Trust your understanding of your child; don't follow a rigid schedule. Have your partner be part of it [by having them] bottle-feed expressed milk during the night so you get more structured sleep."
> —former patient Shirley Qu

CHAPTER 13:

TAKING CARE OF THE MILK-MAKER (THAT'S YOU)

I wish I'd known...

Feeling worse each day *isn't* normal postpartum recovery. It's easy to minimize your own symptoms, telling yourself *I'll be fine* over and over. But every day you should feel a little better, not worse—and if you don't, it's your body telling you something needs medical attention.

In the whirlwind of bringing home a new baby, it's all too easy to put yourself last on the priority list. Between feedings, diaper changes, and trying to figure out why your little one is crying *this* time, many new moms barely have time to shower, let alone check in with their own bodies (but you *must*!).

And I hate to harp on it... but it's a story I hear all too often from moms in my practice: "I thought what I was feeling was normal," or "I didn't want to bother anyone with my problems when the baby needed attention."

Here's the truth: your health matters just as much as your baby's. Not just because you deserve care too (though you absolutely do!), but because your well-being directly impacts your ability to care for your little one. Think of it like those airplane safety demonstrations—you need to put on your own oxygen mask before helping others.

This chapter is your guide to understanding which physical and emotional symptoms deserve immediate attention. Some postpartum changes are completely normal, while others are your body's way of waving a red flag saying "Hey! Something's not right here!" Learning to tell the difference isn't just good self-care—it's essential for your breastfeeding success and your overall experience as a new mother.

So let's talk about what's normal, what's not, and when it's time to pick up the phone and call for help. Because taking care of yourself isn't selfish; it's one of the most important things you can do for your baby.

Birth and Medical Complications

It's estimated that between 14–16% of commercially insured women in the U.S. between the ages of eighteen and forty-four experience a pregnancy or childbirth-related complication. These numbers are often higher in women who have public insurance, such as Medicaid, and who are older than forty-four[60].

I'm not sharing these statistics to scare you—I'm sharing them because knowledge is power. After almost a decade as a labor and delivery nurse, I've seen how birth complications can derail breastfeeding plans when moms aren't prepared. The gap between "I really want to breastfeed" and "But I don't know how to adapt when things get complicated" can be huge.

The good news? Even when birth doesn't go as planned, breastfeeding can still succeed with the right support and strategies. Let's look at some common complications and exactly how to protect your breastfeeding relationship if they happen to you.

Preeclampsia

Preeclampsia is a serious pregnancy complication that can emerge during pregnancy and the postpartum period, impacting both the mother and baby. It affects a notable 5–8% of pregnancies.[61] This condition advances rapidly and is characterized by elevated blood pressure and often the presence of protein in the urine. Beyond these hallmark signs, preeclampsia may manifest in other less obvious symptoms, such as persistent headaches and discomfort in the upper right abdominal area. Recognizing these signs is crucial for early detection and effective management of this condition, potentially safeguarding both maternal and fetal

60 "Trends in Pregnancy and Childbirth Complications in the U.S." Blue Cross Blue Shield, 17 June 2020, www.bcbs.com/the-health-of-america/reports/trends-in-pregnancy-and-childbirth-complications-in-the-us#key-findings.

61 Johns Hopkins Medicine, "Preeclampsia," April 2025.

life and health. Since we are constantly learning new things about preeclampsia, I encourage you to talk with your provider and visit the Preeclampsia Foundation website[62] for the latest information.

Now, how can preeclampsia affect your breastfeeding journey? One word: magnesium. If you have preeclampsia, your medical team might give you a medication called magnesium sulfate (which is totally different from magnesium supplements you might take at home). This medication is extremely helpful for preeclampsia but can have side effects that affect you and your baby—most notably feeling very sleepy, which can make it quite difficult to stay awake to breastfeed. Despite the complications preeclampsia and its treatment can bring to the table, you can still initiate breastfeeding. It just might need a little more patience and understanding.

Here are a few strategies to consider:

1. **Breastfeeding When the Baby's Alert:** Pay close attention to those precious moments when your baby is awake and alert. These are the ideal times to encourage breastfeeding.
2. **Skin-to-Skin Cuddles:** Don't underestimate the power of skin-to-skin contact. It can work wonders for you and your baby, promoting bonding and boosting your milk supply.
3. **Breast Pump Assistance:** If your baby is too drowsy, using a breast pump can help stimulate your milk supply. You can then feed this pumped milk to your baby through a bottle or other feeding methods.
4. **Patience and Support:** Preeclampsia and the effects of the medication used to treat it are usually temporary. Over time, your baby should become more alert and breastfeeding will get easier.

62 www.preeclampsia.org

5. **Consult a Lactation Expert:** Reach out to a lactation consultant or specialist who has experience helping mothers who have dealt with preeclampsia. Their guidance can be invaluable.

Your dedication to providing the best nourishment for your baby while protecting your health is what truly matters. Take a deep breath and remember to take things one week at a time. You've got this! To learn more about preeclampsia, listen to episode 13 of The Boob Business podcast with award-winning obstetrician Dr. Crystal Berry-Roberts.[63]

Postpartum Hemorrhage

Experiencing a postpartum hemorrhage can be terrifying. I've held the hands of moms going through this in my L&D nursing days, and it's definitely not what anyone plans for on their birth day. But remember, you're not alone in this. Let's talk about how this event might affect your breastfeeding plans and how you can prepare for the best possible outcome.

Postpartum hemorrhage, sometimes shortened to PPH, is when a mom goes through heavy bleeding after having her baby (usually losing more than 1,000 milliliters of blood). This typically happens within a day after giving birth, but it can also happen as late as twelve weeks after the baby's arrival. Just like any health challenge, it can leave you feeling both physically and emotionally drained.

After a postpartum hemorrhage you might be at higher risk of having anemia, which can leave you feeling extremely fatigued. It is important to rest and replenish nutrients. Your health and healing should be your top priorities after a big health scare like this. Depending on the severity of the hemorrhage, you might

63 https://www.buzzsprout.com/1885195/episodes/10434066

require some extra care, such as further medical interventions to manage the situation. For instance, your healthcare team might recommend specific medications to help stop the bleeding. In cases of severe hemorrhages, a surgical procedure and possibly a blood transfusion might be necessary. If you are not willing to accept blood from the hospital blood bank if needed to save your life, you will want to discuss this with your midwife or obstetrician during your first or second trimester.

Now, you might be wondering how this event can affect your baby's feeding. Sometimes, a massive loss of blood could affect your body's ability to make larger volumes of milk right away. With proper volume replacement (this is something your doctor would manage with blood transfusions and IV fluids) and proper nutritional support, your body should make a full recovery, including a full milk supply over time.

Once you're stable enough, don't hesitate to advocate for yourself. Request a hospital-issued, commercial-grade breast pump from the medical staff. This device can make a significant difference in stimulating your milk supply, even if you can't breastfeed your baby directly right now. Remember, these early days are what can help set your internal lactation thermostat I mentioned earlier in the book.

Now, let's talk about the emotional side of things. A postpartum hemorrhage can be overwhelming and lead to feelings of anxiety and even trauma. Remember to look after your well-being during this difficult time and rely on the support systems around you. Yes, navigating a postpartum hemorrhage is a challenging experience, but rest assured, you've got what it takes to overcome these hurdles. Trust your healthcare team, embrace your inner strength, and keep your eyes on the prize: your beautiful little one awaiting you.

Maternal Infections

Maternal infections can occur before or during childbirth. They might involve a variety of conditions, from urinary tract infections (UTIs) to more complex issues like chorioamnionitis (a bacterial infection of the amniotic fluid and membranes surrounding the baby). While concerning, this is something your healthcare team is well-prepared to manage. If diagnosed with this infection, you'll likely be administered antibiotics to help fight it. In some cases, you may remain hospitalized for a few extra days to monitor your health and ensure the most effective treatment. If treated promptly and properly, chorioamnionitis should not cause any further complications with your reproductive system or your breast milk supply.

During this time, follow your healthcare provider's recommendations for treatment. Additionally, you *must* rest and allow your body to heal. Don't hesitate to ask questions or voice concerns; your providers are there to guide you and provide the best care possible.

Your baby will also receive thorough evaluation and care. Depending on the situation, your little one might need to spend some time in the NICU. This can be a challenging experience for any parent, but remember, your baby is in good hands, and if this step is taken, it is essential for their health and well-being.

Throughout your treatment, your breast milk will remain a source of nourishment and comfort for your baby. Your healthcare team will help you establish a pumping routine to ensure that you maintain your milk supply. With the right treatment and support from your healthcare team, you and your baby can navigate this stage with strength and resilience.

Diabetes and Breastfeeding

I've worked with so many moms with diabetes who were told breastfeeding might be "too complicated" for them. Let me tell you right now—that's just not true! Yes, there are some unique challenges, but with the right game plan, diabetic moms can absolutely crush their breastfeeding goals. Having diabetes (any form of diabetes) during pregnancy is like running a marathon, where endurance, perseverance, and careful pacing are essential to reach the finish line safely.

If the mother has high blood sugar levels, the baby may be larger than average, which might pose challenges during delivery.[64] It is likely that your provider may recommend inducing your labor early, depending on how quickly your baby is growing. If they are larger than appropriate for their age, your provider will likely want your baby to be born before the full forty weeks. This means that you may give birth to a "normal"-sized baby who is still slightly early. If this is your situation, I highly recommend reading the section "Understanding Preterm Births" in chapter 14.

Additionally, some babies born to diabetic mothers might have low blood sugar levels initially, which means they may need to be fed more frequently. Babies of diabetic mothers can struggle with blood sugar regulation during the early days, making breastfeeding more complex. If your baby was born larger due to your diabetes, they might need more colostrum than you can produce. Additionally, some diabetic women may take longer to produce enough milk,[65] putting them at risk for low supply. But these challenges don't mean you can't breastfeed; they just mean you might need extra strategies.

---

64 National Institutes of Health (NIH), "Mothers' High Normal Blood Sugar Levels Place Infants at Risk for Birth Problems," May 7, 2008.

65 PubMed Central, "Hypoglycemia and Associated Comorbidities Among Newborns of Mothers with Diabetes Mellitus," October 13, 2023.

The good news is that breastfeeding can help manage your blood sugar levels.[66] Your breast milk is also designed to provide consistent nourishment and stabilize your baby's sugar levels. Colostrum is particularly helpful for this.

While we've covered complications that might arise during birth, many postpartum issues can develop in the days and weeks after you're home with your baby. This is when you're likely to be most focused on your little one and might miss signs that your body needs attention too. Let's break down the most common physical warning signs that mean it's time to call your healthcare provider—because sometimes, knowing when to make that call can make all the difference.

Postpartum Warning Signs

After giving birth, your body goes through incredible changes as it recovers and adapts to breastfeeding. Most discomforts during this time are normal parts of healing, but some symptoms deserve immediate attention. As someone who ignored her own warning signs (big mistake!), I want to help you recognize when something needs medical care versus when it's just part of the normal postpartum journey.

Let's break down the most common physical warning signs that mean it's time to call your healthcare provider. These aren't meant to scare you—they're meant to empower you with information so you can advocate for yourself. Because sometimes, the difference between a minor issue and a serious complication is simply how quickly you get help.

---

66 Kaiser Permanente Division of Research, "Fully or Mostly Breastfeeding Women Have Lowest Blood Sugar Levels After a Gestational Diabetes Pregnancy," April 2025.

Fever or Chills

You have a slightly higher risk of infections in the postpartum period.[67] Uterine infections, urinary tract infections, and perineal infections can occur. While it's not uncommon to experience a mild post-birth fever due to hormonal changes,[68] persistent fever or chills should be taken seriously. Infections don't happen often but may lead to severe complications if left untreated. Timely diagnosis and treatment are essential. A fever in an adult is considered an oral temperature of 100.4°F (38°C) or above.[69]

Here's what I've seen happen too many times: new moms get so focused on their baby's health that they completely minimize their own symptoms. "I'll be fine, I'll be fine," you tell yourself while something serious develops under the surface. Remember that while you were in the hospital, you were likely getting regular doses of pain medication (at least 600 milligrams of ibuprofen), which can mask a fever. That's why these symptoms often don't show up until you're home. So listen up: if you experience chills—which usually come before a fever—take your temperature immediately. Don't wait, don't second-guess, and definitely don't brush it off as "just being tired." This isn't being dramatic; it's being your own best advocate when your body is trying to tell you something important.

Red Streak on One Breast with Fever and Chills

If you observe a red streak on one of your breasts and experience fever and chills, it could indicate mastitis. Mastitis occurs in approximately 10% of breastfeeding women[70] and usually affects just one breast.

---

67 Merck Manuals, "Infections of the Uterus After Delivery," August 7, 2024.

68 Lecturio, "Postpartum Fever," February 16, 2023.

69 MedlinePlus, "Body Temperature Norms: MedlinePlus Medical Encyclopedia," February 2, 2023.

70 PubMed Central, "Management of Mastitis in Breastfeeding Women," September 15, 2008.

I want to share some important insights from Dr. Katrina Mitchell,[71] a board-certified breast surgeon and IBCLC who specializes in this area. Mastitis is essentially a painful inflammation of breast tissue that causes symptoms like swelling, redness, fever, chills, and general discomfort.

In my own practice, I've found that what many moms don't realize is that mastitis is rarely an infection—it's actually an inflammatory condition. It's typically caused by oversupply or temporary engorgement in a specific area of breast tissue. Those "milk sacs" (the alveolar cells) become painful and lumpy, while increased blood flow makes the area red and swollen.

For more information on mastitis and how to treat it, see the Resources section in the back of this book.

And please note: it is advised to call your doctor anytime you get a fever.

Excessive Bleeding

Bleeding after childbirth, known as lochia, is a normal part of the post-birth process, but it can sometimes indicate a more serious issue. If you experience heavy bleeding with large clots, it might suggest retained placenta, where parts of the placenta remain in the uterus. This can prevent your uterus from contracting properly to control bleeding, which can also contribute to an infection in your uterus. You should also know if any part of the placenta remains in the uterus it can completely inhibit milk production until it is completely removed.[72] Early detection and treatment are crucial.

---

71 https://physicianguidetobreastfeeding.org/about-the-physician/

72 PubMed, "Disruption of Lactogenesis by Retained Placental Fragments," February 2002.

Persistent Headache, Blurred Vision, or Upper Right Abdominal Pain

Postpartum headaches are quite common and can often be attributed to hormonal changes, fatigue, or dehydration. However, a persistent or severe headache, especially when accompanied by abdominal pain or visual disturbances like spots or blurring, could be a sign of postpartum preeclampsia. Refer back to the "Preeclampsia" section of this chapter.

When to Call for Help

If you experience any of these signs or are concerned about your postpartum health, reach out to your healthcare provider. Early intervention and appropriate care are essential to ensure a smooth transition into motherhood.

Nine Key Postpartum Warning Signs

Below is a list of nine post-birth warning signs created by the Association of Women's Health, Obstetric and Neonatal Nurses (AWHONN) in 2023. They can signal serious complications and ignoring them can lead to life-threatening emergencies. Seek immediate medical attention if you experience *any* of these symptoms:

- ☐ P - Pain in chest
- ☐ O - Obstructed breathing or shortness of breath
- ☐ S - Seizures
- ☐ T - Thoughts of hurting yourself or someone else
- ☐ B - Bleeding, soaking through one pad an hour, or large clots
- ☐ I - Incision that isn't healing
- ☐ R - Red, swollen leg that's painful or warm to the touch
- ☐ T - Temperature of 100.4°F (38°C) or higher or 96.8°F (36°C) or lower (a possible sign of infection/sepsis)
- ☐ H - Headache that doesn't go away with medication or vision changes

To learn more, listen to episode 45 of The Boob Business Podcast.[73]

Mental and Emotional Health: Recognizing When It's More Than Just Baby Blues

While it's perfectly normal to experience occasional stress and worry as a new mom, it's essential to differentiate between typical emotions and potential signs of more serious conditions like postpartum anxiety or depression.

Here are tips to ensure your emotional well-being during this time:

1. **Know Yourself:** Take time to identify what specifically triggers anxiety or depression for you. For some, it's sleep deprivation. For others, it's the pressure to breastfeed flawlessly.

73 https://www.buzzsprout.com/1885195/episodes/16738158

2. **Keep a Journal:** Writing about your experiences can help you uncover recurring sources of stress or sadness. Daily reflections may reveal patterns that highlight areas where you could use extra support.
3. **Seek Support:** Always remember the positives of seeking help. If you spot any signs of postpartum anxiety or depression, or if you're feeling overwhelmed, reach out to a perinatal mental health counselor. They're equipped to offer emotional support and provide treatment for women and couples facing challenges during pregnancy, birth, and early stage parenting. Remember that you're not alone on this journey.

Call or text the National Maternal Mental Health Hotline at 1-833-TLC-MAMA for free mental health support. Reach out anytime you feel overwhelmed, anxious, or just need someone to talk to. It is completely free!

If you ever have thoughts of harming yourself or your baby, this is an emergency—please call or text 988 (the Suicide and Crisis Lifeline) or go to your nearest emergency room (ER) immediately. Don't wait, don't second-guess, and don't try to handle these feelings alone.

Not sure if what you're feeling is "normal" or something more serious? The Edinburgh Postnatal Depression Scale (EPDS) is a simple self-assessment that can help you determine if you might be experiencing postpartum depression or anxiety. You can find it online[74], and it takes just a few minutes to complete. While it's not a diagnostic tool, bringing your completed questionnaire to your healthcare provider can be incredibly helpful in starting that important conversation.

---

74 https://med.stanford.edu/content/dam/sm/neonatology/documents/edinburghscale.pdf

Remember that you're not alone on this journey—many mothers experience these challenges, and effective help is available.

When to Talk to Your Doctor

Here are some other signals that it might be time for a chat with a healthcare provider:

- **Persistent Feelings:** If feelings of anxiety, sadness, or despair persist beyond the first few weeks, it's essential to seek help.
- **Disrupting Daily Life:** When these emotions start interfering with your daily life and your ability to care for yourself or your baby, it's time to reach out.
- **Physical Symptoms:** Sometimes, postpartum mood disorders can manifest with physical symptoms, such as changes in appetite or sleep patterns. If these accompany emotional changes, it's time to seek assistance.
- **Intense Worries:** If you find yourself overwhelmed by fears regarding your baby's well-being, even when everything is fine, it's important to talk to a healthcare professional.

Please know that dads and partners can also experience postpartum depression. At least one in seven women and one in ten men suffer from postpartum depression.[75] Postpartum Support International has wonderful resources if you suspect you or your partner are struggling with a postpartum mood disorder.

Also, be sure to listen to episode 23 of The Boob Business Podcast[76] to learn more about the signs and symptoms of postpartum mood disorders.

75 UnityPoint Health, "Male Postpartum Depression," April 2025.

76 https://www.buzzsprout.com/1885195/episodes/12635187

Finding Your Flow: Becoming Your Own Advocate

Finding your flow when dealing with postpartum complications means becoming your own best advocate. I see moms ignore their own symptoms all the time in my practice—I did it myself! But remember this: caring for yourself isn't taking away from caring for your baby; it's ensuring you'll be there for them in the best possible health. Trust your instincts when something feels wrong. Pay attention to the warning signs we've discussed. And most importantly, don't hesitate to reach out for help. Whether that's calling your provider about a persistent headache or connecting with a mental health professional when the baby blues don't lift, speaking up is the first step toward healing. Your baby needs you healthy and whole, not silently struggling through complications that could be managed with proper care. This is the time to find your voice along with your flow—both are essential to your journey as a new mother. You've got this, mama!

Mom-to-Mom Insight: "I wish I would have known how much of a mental load would accompany breastfeeding and pumping. The learning curve is so high for a new mom, on top of caring for a baby while exhausted. Once I finally got the hang of nursing, had the right pumping supplies, and figured out why flange sizes were so important, I was still consumed by continually tracking ounces, wondering if my food choices were why my baby was having tummy issues, cleaning never-ending pump and bottle parts, and questioning if my milk supply was sufficient. Though it all has been worth it, there have been times the journey was very isolating." —former patient Ashley Weatherly

CHAPTER 14:

KEEPING YOUR LITTLE ONE SAFE AND THRIVING

I wish I'd known...

Bringing your baby home doesn't require a medical degree. It requires knowing which signs actually matter. You don't need to catch every little hiccup and grunt. You just need to be aware of the real warning signs so you can spot them if they should happen... while *also* giving yourself permission to sleep when you can.

Those first days at home with your tiny human can feel like a crash course in newborn detective work. Is that grunting normal? Should their poop really be that color? What's with all the hiccups?

Let me first put your mind at ease: most of those little quirks are completely normal. But there are some specific signs that genuinely deserve your attention—ones that help you know when your baby might need extra support with feeding or when it's time to call your healthcare provider.

Birth-Related Medical Complications

When a baby faces medical challenges from birth, it can certainly impact your breastfeeding journey—but that doesn't mean breastfeeding isn't possible. Understanding what's happening with your baby and how to adapt is key to providing your milk despite these hurdles. Let's look at some common birth-related complications and specific strategies to protect your breastfeeding relationship through each one.

Understanding Preterm Births: A Precious Start to the Journey

Preterm babies are those born before thirty-seven weeks of gestation. In the United States, about one in ten babies arrives early.[77] These little warriors arrive into the world earlier than expected, bringing unique challenges with them. They haven't had the same time to develop within the womb, so they typically lack the endurance and stamina to feed effectively. This doesn't mean they won't get there; it just means it might take more time. Imagine preparing for a marathon—you wouldn't expect to run one straight out of the gate. Similarly, a baby born at thirty-

77 Centers for Disease Control and Prevention, "Preterm Birth," Maternal and Infant Health, last modified February 24, 2025, accessed April 8, 2025, https://www.cdc.gov/maternal-infant-health/preterm-birth/index.html.

seven weeks might need a few weeks to develop the stamina for exclusive breastfeeding.

Here's the biggest challenge: babies usually can't properly coordinate sucking, swallowing, and breathing until after thirty-nine weeks of gestation. Many babies born after thirty-nine to forty weeks can master this coordination from scratch.[78] Some preterm babies might need help from a feeding tube and guidance from a pediatric feeding therapist—often occupational therapists or speech language therapists who help fine-tune these skills.

Don't rush this natural process. Every baby has a unique timeline for learning these skills. I'd actually advise against expecting your little one to perform the dance of exclusive breastfeeding in the early weeks. Instead, adopt a flexible approach that meets your baby's daily needs. For preterm babies especially, working with a lactation consultant is invaluable—they'll be your guiding star as your baby develops the skills needed for successful breastfeeding.

Navigating Jaundice in Newborns

Jaundice is a common condition in newborns that causes a yellowish tint to appear on a baby's skin and eyes—though this coloring can be harder to detect in babies with darker skin tones. As I learned with my own son, the yellowing might not be obvious until it reaches the whites of the eyes, especially in babies with olive, brown, or black skin. This happens when bilirubin, a yellow pigment, builds up in their blood. Your baby's liver is still developing, so it may not be able to process bilirubin as efficiently as an adult's liver. Several factors can contribute to an increase in bilirubin levels, including significant bruising to the baby from birth trauma or when the mother and baby have different blood types. Additionally, babies of Asian descent tend to have higher

78 PubMed Central, "Oral and Respiratory Control for Preterm Feeding," July 2008.

rates of jaundice.[79] Babies are usually tested for jaundice between twenty-four to thirty-six hours of life.

The Sleepiness Challenge

Jaundice creates a challenging cycle for breastfeeding: the condition makes babies extra sleepy and less interested in feeding, but frequent feeding is exactly what helps reduce jaundice by increasing bowel movements that eliminate bilirubin. When my first son had jaundice, I felt like I was constantly trying to wake a peacefully sleeping baby who needed to eat but wouldn't stay awake to do it!

The best way to manage jaundice is through a combination of approaches:

- Feed your baby frequently using breastfeeding, hand expression, and/or supplementing with donor breast milk if needed. (For supplementing techniques that protect breastfeeding, see chapter 11.)
- Engage in skin-to-skin contact to help keep your baby awake and attentive during feeds.
- If your baby is too sleepy to breastfeed effectively, consider pumping and supplementing with expressed milk to ensure adequate nourishment.
- Don't miss follow-up appointments to monitor bilirubin levels.
- If jaundice becomes severe, treatments like phototherapy (special lights that break down bilirubin) are available.

Jaundice is just a temporary bump on your breastfeeding path, not a roadblock. With your commitment to breastfeeding and the support of your healthcare team, you can help your baby navigate

79 PubMed Central, "Neonatal Jaundice in Asian, White, and Mixed-Race Infants," March 5, 2002

jaundice-related sleepiness and keep the breastfeeding journey bright and clear. Brighter days are on the way!

Breathing Challenges: Respiratory Distress Syndrome

One obstacle many premature babies encounter is respiratory distress syndrome (RDS). This condition can arise for multiple reasons, including underdeveloped lungs, infection, or aspiration, creating breathing challenges that often need specialized care.

In the face of RDS, providing your milk to your baby remains incredibly important. Here's how to navigate breastfeeding during this challenge:

- **Advocate for Kangaroo Care:** Placing your baby skin-to-skin on your chest stabilizes vital signs, promotes milk supply,[80] and strengthens your bond.
- **Initiate Early Pumping:** Since direct latching might not be immediately feasible, expressing milk is vital. The NICU staff will help establish an effective pumping schedule.
- **Store Milk Properly:** Your expressed breast milk can be stored for your baby's feedings. The NICU team will guide you on appropriate storage and labeling procedures.
- **Adapt to Feeding Methods:** Depending on your baby's condition, they may initially require feeding via a feeding tube or bottle. You can still provide kangaroo care and work on latching when your baby is ready.
- **Work with the NICU Team:** Communicate your breastfeeding goals clearly and follow their guidance on when to attempt direct breastfeeding.

80 HealthyChildren.org, "Skin-to-Skin Contact: How Kangaroo Care Benefits Your Baby," April 2025.

As challenging as RDS can be, remember that your milk provides both comfort and essential nourishment for your baby as their tiny lungs develop strength. Your commitment makes a difference, even when the journey looks different than expected.

Newborn Infections: Safeguarding Breastfeeding

One of motherhood's unexpected challenges can emerge when your newborn faces infections like sepsis, pneumonia, or urinary tract infections. Here's how to maintain your breastfeeding journey while supporting your baby through these medical situations.

Types of Newborn Infections:

1. **Sepsis:** Sepsis is a full-body infection in newborns that requires immediate medical attention. Sometimes, this means your baby might be separated from you for treatment. During this time, you can use a breast pump to express milk. This keeps your milk flowing while your little one gets the care they need.
2. **Pneumonia:** Pneumonia can make breathing a bit tricky for your baby. It might affect nursing, and that's when the experts can step in to help you figure out the safest way to feed your little champ. Be sure to follow the guidance of your doctors and lactation consultant to address the needs of your baby's situation.
3. **Urinary Tract Infections:** UTIs aren't very common in newborns. If your baby does get one, they might appear fussier during feeds and will typically have a fever. Luckily, most UTIs can be treated with antibiotics, and your baby should be able to continue breastfeeding normally. Again, contact your medical provider any time your baby gets a fever.

Strategies for Breastfeeding Babies with Infections:

1. **Talk to the Healthcare Team:** Your medical team will be your go-to source for dealing with these infections. They'll provide the best advice on how to handle feeding and ensure your baby stays safe and recovers.
2. **Pump and Store:** If you must be separated from your baby due to a severe infection like sepsis, a breast pump will be your new BFF. It helps maintain your milk supply and ensures your baby still gets all those fantastic breast milk benefits.
3. **Prioritize Comfort and Bonding:** In tough times, embrace skin-to-skin contact and gentle touches. They're a wonderful way to stay connected with your baby during these challenges, and they provide comfort for both of you.

Remember that each newborn infection situation is unique, and your medical team is there to guide you with treatments catered toward your baby's specific needs. Don't be shy in sharing your concerns and asking questions. Your determination to breastfeed, even in the face of unexpected medical issues, reflects your love and care for your newborn.

Feeding Warning Signs

While birth complications like jaundice or preterm delivery can certainly impact feeding, even babies born without these challenges can struggle to get enough milk. As new parents, we're often told to trust our instincts, but how do you develop those instincts when everything about having a newborn is new to you?

In my practice, I've found that parents who know exactly what to look for feel much more confident than those trying to navigate by guesswork. Let's look at some specific, observable signs that help you know when your baby is getting enough to eat—and when they might need additional support. Think of these as your breastfeeding navigation tools, helping you spot potential issues before they become bigger problems:

Signs Baby Isn't Getting Enough Milk

When parents ask me how they can tell if their baby is getting enough milk, I tell them to look for these four key indicators:

1. Listen for Swallowing Sounds

One of the most reassuring sounds during breastfeeding is your baby's gentle, rhythmic swallows. It's like a little "Ka, ka" that lets you know they're actively transferring milk. Not every suck equals a swallow, though—effective feeding typically shows a pattern where your baby sucks several times and then you hear that distinct swallow. If you're rarely or never hearing these swallows, particularly after your milk has come in around days three to five, it could indicate your baby isn't getting enough milk.

2. Watch Post-Feed Behavior

A well-fed baby usually shows a distinct "milk-drunk" contentment after feeding. They might drift off to sleep with relaxed hands and a peaceful expression or stay calmly awake. If your baby consistently remains fussy, continues rooting or showing hunger cues immediately after feeding, or seems frustrated at the breast, these behaviors suggest they may not be getting enough to satisfy them. The occasional fussy feed is normal, but a pattern of dissatisfaction after most feeds deserves attention.

3. Count Those Wet Diapers

Your baby's diaper output is like a built-in hydration gauge. After your milk comes in, expect about six to eight wet diapers per day.

The urine should be pale yellow—like diluted lemonade—not dark or concentrated. If you notice reddish-brown "brick dust" in their diaper, call your provider right away, as this suggests significant dehydration.

4. Track Weight Patterns

Weight gain is perhaps the most objective measure of feeding success. While a 5–7 percent weight loss is normal in the first few days, your baby should start regaining weight after your milk comes in and be back to birth weight by ten to fourteen days. After that, expect your baby to gain about an ounce per day for the first three months.[81] If your baby isn't regaining weight as expected or is still losing weight after day five, it's time to get help from a lactation professional.

> **Rule of Thumb:** One bad day isn't a crisis, but patterns matter. If your baby is experiencing one of these warning signs for more than one or two days, reach out to a lactation consultant or your pediatrician rather than waiting to see if things improve.

5. Lack of Interest

If your baby is consistently drowsy or uninterested in feeding, it could signal a problem. Babies typically approach feeding time with enthusiasm—it's their favorite activity! But when they suddenly seem disinterested or too sleepy to eat, it's like when you're so exhausted you can't enjoy your favorite meal.

When this pattern persists for more than twenty-four hours, something might be making your baby too sleepy to feed effectively. This requires attention from a healthcare professional

81 Nemours KidsHealth, "Your Newborn's Growth," January 16, 2024.

who can determine the cause of the lethargy and help restore your baby's natural feeding patterns. Seek professional help with this issue, as maintaining proper nutrition is essential for your baby's development.

Stooling Patterns and Concerns

Your baby's diapers tell an important story about their feeding success and overall health. Learning to read these diaper messages means knowing what's normal and what needs attention.

Normal Stool Development

During the first week, your baby's stool will transform dramatically[82]:

- **Days 1–2**: Expect meconium—that dark, greenish-black, sticky substance that looks like tar. This is completely normal and is your baby's first bowel movement.
- **Days 3–4**: As your milk comes in, you'll see transitional stools—a mix of meconium and milk stool that appears brownish-green.
- **Days 5+**: Once your mature milk is well-established, breastfed babies typically have yellow, seedy stools with the consistency of mustard. Some describe it as looking like little yellow seeds in a yellow sauce.

Normal Stooling Frequency

Newborns between one week and six weeks of life usually stool more than five times per day. This frequent stooling is a good sign—it indicates your baby is getting plenty of milk and their digestive system is working well. Some babies may even stool with nearly every feeding in the early weeks! As they get older (around

82 Children's Hospital of Philadelphia (CHOP), "The Scoop on Infant Poop: Is That Normal?" April 2025

six to eight weeks), some exclusively breastfed babies may reduce frequency to once every few days, which can be normal if the baby is gaining weight well.[83]

Warning Signs in Stool Patterns

Pay attention to these changes that might indicate a feeding or health concern:

- **Sudden Decrease in Frequency**: If your well-established baby suddenly stops having regular bowel movements, especially during the first month, this could signal they're not getting enough milk. This pattern change deserves prompt attention from your healthcare provider or lactation consultant.
- **Red Streaks**: Small red streaks occasionally appear from minor rectal irritation and are usually nothing to worry about. However, more pronounced or persistent bleeding needs medical evaluation.
- **Black, Tarry Stools** (after day three): While normal in the first few days, black stools that return later can indicate blood higher in the digestive tract. These stools look like sticky, black coffee grounds and require immediate medical attention.
- **Pale or White Stools**: These chalky-colored stools can signal liver or gallbladder problems, as they suggest a lack of bile needed for fat digestion. Call your healthcare provider right away if you notice this unusual color.
- **Watery, Frequent Stools**: While breastfed baby poop is normally loose, extremely watery stools that seem excessive may indicate diarrhea, which can quickly lead to dehydration in a newborn.

83 La Leche League International, "Constipation," September 25, 2023.

> **Rule of Thumb:** A picture is worth a thousand words when it comes to unusual baby poop. When in doubt, snap a photo of concerning diapers before disposing of them. This visual information can be invaluable to your healthcare provider.

Understanding these stool patterns helps you monitor your baby's health and provides valuable information about their feeding success. Minor color variations are normal, but significant changes should prompt a conversation with your healthcare provider.

Digestive Concerns: Spit-Up, Vomiting, and Diarrhea

Babies spit up, but if it's happening a lot, or if they have diarrhea, it's a concern. Let me help you understand when to be concerned and when to know things are normal.

Spit-Up

When a baby spits up, it's usually a gentle flow of stomach contents coming back up, often right after feeding. It's kind of like when you fill your glass too quickly with water from the tap and it overflows slightly. Spit-up is usually effortless, and it doesn't seem to bother your baby much. It's quite common, and many babies do it. In some European countries, parents refer to this as "spilling." If your baby is spitting up occasionally, it's usually not a cause for concern. However, if the spitting up is frequent, forceful, or accompanied by other signs of discomfort like fussiness or weight loss, it's a good idea to consult your healthcare provider.

Vomiting

Vomiting is more forceful and can look quite different from spit-up. It's when your baby uses their abdominal muscles to forcefully expel their stomach contents—it's a much stronger and more noticeable event than a gentle stream of spit-up. Vomiting can be concerning because it might be a sign of an underlying issue, like an infection or a blockage.

Diarrhea

Diarrhea in a baby is like a faucet that's been turned on too high, and water is gushing out rapidly, unlike the usual slow stream you expect. It means your baby is passing loose, watery stools more frequently than usual. Diarrhea can lead to dehydration, especially in babies, as they lose fluids and important electrolytes quickly. If your baby is experiencing frequent vomiting or diarrhea, it's essential to reach out to a healthcare professional. They can help identify the cause and provide guidance on how to keep your little one hydrated and comfortable.

Poor Latch as a Feeding Warning Sign

It's important to recognize when a poor latch is affecting your baby's ability to get enough milk. Watch for these baby-focused warning signs:

- Your baby repeatedly pulls away from the breast frustrated or crying.
- You notice your baby's cheeks dimpling or hear clicking sounds during feeds.
- Your baby seems to be working hard but not satisfying their hunger.
- Weight gain slows despite frequent feeding attempts.

These signs suggest your baby may not be extracting milk efficiently, even if they appear to be nursing often. If you notice these patterns, especially alongside other warning signs like decreased wet diapers or slow weight gain, it's time to revisit chapter 9 and consult with a lactation professional who can help improve your baby's milk transfer.

Urgent Warning Signs: When to Get Immediate Help

While feeding challenges need attention, there are certain warning signs that deserve a faster response—the kind where you don't wait until morning or your next scheduled appointment. These are the situations where your mama bear instincts should kick into high gear. As always, I'm not sharing these to scare you but to empower you with knowledge that could make all the difference in an emergency situation. Now, before you start worrying, keep in mind: most babies will never experience these issues. But just like it's good to know cardiopulmonary resuscitation even while hoping you'll never need to use it, recognizing these urgent warning signs means you'll be prepared to act quickly if they ever appear. Let's walk through the situations that warrant immediate medical attention:

Breathing Problems

If your baby is breathing too fast (more than sixty breaths per minute)[84] or showing signs of respiratory distress, take immediate action. Warning signs include flaring nostrils, whistling or high-pitched humming sounds with each breath, and visible chest retractions where the skin pulls in between or below the ribs.

A baby struggling to breathe will likely be unable to breastfeed properly. This rapid, labored breathing indicates they're working too hard for something that should come naturally. This is a serious red flag that might suggest issues with their lungs, airways, or heart.

84 Cleveland Clinic, "Jaundice in Newborns: Symptoms, Causes & Treatment," March 19, 2025

Seek emergency help—breathing difficulties are never a wait-and-see situation, and prompt medical attention can make all the difference for your baby's health.

Action: Seek immediate emergency care (call 911) if your baby is having breathing difficulties.

Newborn Fevers

A fever in a newborn is a significant red flag. Their little bodies can't fight infections effectively yet, which makes any temperature elevation potentially serious. As a rule, an oral temperature of 99.4°F or higher is considered a fever and requires immediate medical attention.[85]

Never attempt to lower a newborn's fever with over-the-counter medication without consulting your healthcare provider first. Their guidance is essential for your baby's safety. This is one symptom where prompt medical evaluation is always warranted, regardless of how well your baby might otherwise appear.

Action: Seek immediate emergency care (call 911 or go to the ER) if your baby has an oral temperature of 99.4°F or higher.

Color Changes

Babies are usually a bit pale when they're born, and each baby has their own unique and beautiful shades, reflecting their heritage. But if you notice their colors fading, turning unusually pale, gray, or bluish, it's a clear sign that something might be affecting their breathing or circulation. Regardless of your baby's ethnicity, significant or persistent changes in their natural skin color should be taken seriously. It's a universal warning sign of a potential issue with oxygen in their body. This is not a wait-and-see situation.

85 Mayo Clinic Health System, "Recognize & Respond to Infant Fevers," April 2025.

Action: Seek immediate emergency care (call 911 or go to the ER) if your baby has become blue, gray, or very pale.

Seizures

Unusual movements, staring spells, or twitching can be signs of seizures in babies. Think of a seizure as an electrical disturbance in your baby's brain—like someone briefly turning off the playground lights, causing all activity to freeze or become chaotic.

Your baby might jerk repeatedly, stare blankly, or make unusual movements that don't respond to your voice or touch. These movements aren't voluntary and often follow a pattern. Seizures signal that something needs attention in your baby's developing brain, and immediate medical evaluation is essential. If you suspect your baby is having a seizure, this is *always* an emergency requiring prompt medical care. This is not a wait-and-see situation.

Action: Seek immediate emergency care (call 911 or go to the ER) if your baby is experiencing a seizure or making unusual jerking movements.

Dehydration Signs

Dehydration means your baby's body doesn't have enough fluids to work properly. Watch for these warning signs:

- **Sunken Soft Spot:** Sinking or depression in the soft spot (fontanel) on top of your baby's head
- **Dry Mouth:** Parched lips and mouth with little or no saliva
- **Dark Urine:** Orange or rust-colored urine in diapers
- **Lack of Tears:** Crying without producing tears
- **Weak Cry:** Unusually faint or whisper-like crying sounds
- **Lethargy:** Excessive sleepiness, difficulty waking, or unusual lack of responsiveness

Dehydration can occur from fever, diarrhea, or insufficient milk intake. Babies dehydrate quickly due to their small size, which is why frequent feedings are essential. If you notice these signs, contact your doctor immediately. This is not a wait-and-see situation.

Important: If you suspect dehydration, *do not* give your baby water unless directed by your baby's doctor.

Action: Seek immediate emergency care (call 911 or go to the ER) if your baby is showing signs of dehydration.

Physical Responses: Stiffness or Floppiness:
If your baby's muscle tone seems unusual—either too floppy or too stiff—it could indicate a problem requiring medical attention.

Healthy newborns have balanced muscle tone that allows them to move naturally while maintaining some position control. When holding your baby, you should feel some resistance in their limbs—not complete limpness like a rag doll, nor rigid stiffness that resists gentle movement.

"Too floppy" means your baby feels limp with little muscle resistance when moved, while "too stiff" means their limbs resist normal bending and seem constantly tense. Either extreme could signal neurological or muscular issues that need prompt medical evaluation. Trust your instincts if your baby's muscle tone doesn't feel right. This is not a wait-and-see situation.

Action: Seek immediate emergency care (call 911 or go to the ER) if your baby is showing signs of extreme floppiness or stiffness.

Response Guide: When to Act and How

While all the warning signs we've discussed deserve attention, knowing how quickly to respond can be just as important as recognizing the sign itself. Here's a quick reference guide:

Get Emergency Care Immediately (Call 911 or Go to the ER):

- Breathing problems (rapid breathing, flaring nostrils, retractions, grunting)
- Blue or gray color, especially around the lips
- Seizures or unusual jerking movements
- Severe dehydration with lethargy and sunken fontanel
- Extreme floppiness or unresponsiveness
- Fever in babies under eight weeks (100.4°F/38°C or higher)

Call Your Doctor Today:

- Moderate signs of dehydration (decreased wet diapers, darker urine)
- Unusual skin color changes that aren't blue or gray
- Yellow skin/eyes that appears to be worsening
- Excessive vomiting (more than occasional spit-up)
- Persistent diarrhea
- Significant changes in feeding patterns with other symptoms

Discuss at Your Next Appointment:

- Minor changes in stool color (without other symptoms)
- Occasional fussiness after feeds (without weight loss)
- Mild spit-up that doesn't bother your baby
- Questions about normal developmental changes

Remember, you know your baby best. If something feels wrong, don't hesitate to seek help, even if the symptoms don't exactly match these categories. It's always better to make a call that turns out to be unnecessary than to miss something important because you were trying not to overreact. Trust those parental instincts—they're usually right!

Finding Your Flow: Vigilance Without Anxiety

Your breastfeeding journey is strong and adaptable, just like you and your precious baby. While infant complications might throw some curveballs, they don't have to knock you off your breastfeeding journey. With some determination, patience, and the right medical guidance, you can handle these hurdles and give your baby the nourishment and comfort that breastfeeding brings. Understanding infant complications sets the stage for informed choices and empowers you to stand up for the best possible breastfeeding experience, even when life throws unexpected challenges your way. Parenthood is a journey full of surprises, but your love and dedication will always light the way.

Mom-to-Mom Insight: "If you feel like something is wrong, advocate for yourself and your baby, even if that means firing and finding new providers and researching the heck out of who will provide you answers. Breastfeeding is hard enough, and complications alongside breastfeeding, like oral restrictions, can seem like the end of your breastfeeding journey, and there were many times I wanted to throw in the towel. Ask for help, dig for answers, ask questions—and if you are able to find and surround yourself with a supportive team of lactation and oral restriction experts, they will advocate for you too."
—former patient Angela Flowers

CHAPTER 15:

BEYOND SURVIVAL MODE TO FINDING YOUR FLOW

I wish I'd known...

The most confident moms aren't the ones who get everything right from day one. They're the ones who learn to trust their instincts and aren't afraid to rewrite their feeding plan.

Those first intense weeks with your baby are behind you, and you're entering a new phase of your breastfeeding journey. This is typically when the initial fog of newborn care begins to lift, and you start asking questions about your long-term feeding approach. Should you pump? Bottle-feed? Exclusively breastfeed? Mix approaches? All these questions are completely normal at this stage.

Around this time, many parents naturally begin making adjustments to their original feeding plans. Reality has a way of reshaping our expectations. You might be craving more flexibility to get out of the house or have your partner take some feedings. Perhaps your partner is returning to work, leaving you to manage feeds alone. Or you might be experiencing that isolation many new mothers feel—what experts call "the invisible pain of postpartum."[86]

> **Rule of Thumb:** Your feeding plan isn't set in stone. The ability to adapt and adjust as you and your baby grow together is a strength, not a failure. Give yourself permission to evolve.

The most important thing to understand is that finding your flow with feeding takes time. Just like learning any new skill, breastfeeding has a learning curve for both you and your baby. Unlike other skills where you might have months to practice and perfect your technique, breastfeeding happens in real-time with real consequences: a hungry baby needs to eat now, not after you've mastered the perfect latch.

But try not to worry. You don't need to have everything figured out immediately. The ideal feeding approach for your family will

86 Blue Cross Blue Shield of Michigan, "Isolation and Loneliness Among New Mothers Can Lead to Postpartum Anxiety and Depression," May 4, 2024

emerge gradually as you both learn and grow together. Most mothers find that around the eight-week mark, patterns begin to take shape and confidence builds. Until then, patience with yourself is just as important as patience with your baby.

During this transition time, common concerns like spit-up, gas, and reflux often become focal points. It's tempting to search online for solutions or worry that something is wrong with your milk or technique. What's hard for many parents to accept is that these issues are usually normal parts of infant development. Your baby's digestive system is maturing alongside everything else. Understanding this won't necessarily make these challenges less stressful, but it might help you worry a bit less about your breastfeeding abilities.

Milestones and Improvements to Celebrate

When I look back at my own journey and those of the thousands of moms I've worked with, I see clear patterns of progress that show you're moving forward. Let me share some of those victories to watch for:

Physical and Practical Achievements:

- ✓ The first time you leave the house alone with your baby
- ✓ The first time you successfully feed your baby somewhere other than your house
- ✓ Sleeping solidly for four to six hours overnight

Feeding Victories:

- ✓ Experiencing decreased pain with nursing or no pain at all
- ✓ Noticing your baby being consistently satisfied after feeding

- ✓ Hearing and identifying swallowing sounds regularly
- ✓ Having more milk-drunk, happy baby moments throughout the day
- ✓ Reducing latch time from perhaps thirty minutes to just ten to fifteen minutes
- ✓ Being able to nurse in multiple positions instead of just one

System Improvements:

- ✓ Becoming more confident in reading your baby's cues
- ✓ Feeding schedules becoming more predictable
- ✓ Getting better at distinguishing between hunger cues and sleep cues
- ✓ Gas symptoms and spit-up usually improving
- ✓ Being able to start shaping your baby's schedule a bit

However, it's important to remember that in those first eight to twelve weeks, your feeding journey is like the stock market—it's all over the place and very unpredictable. After eight to twelve weeks, you can usually start predicting and helping shape your baby's schedule more effectively.

The Mindset Shift: Drawing Your Own Picture

The biggest change I notice in moms during this transition isn't just about the physical aspects of feeding—it's about mindset. The most important shift happens when you start letting go of the Instagram-perfect picture and instead get comfortable drawing your own picture of what your breastfeeding journey is going to look like. This isn't about perfection—it's about progress. You need to pace yourself, celebrate all wins, and know that this takes time. Your journey isn't going to be resolved in the next five days, and that's okay. Let me share some real examples of what finding your flow can look like:

I had a mom who initially planned to exclusively breastfeed. As she approached six to eight weeks, she realized that for her mental health and happiness, she felt better breastfeeding in the morning when things were chill at her house, then switching to pumping and bottle-feeding in the afternoon when her other kid and husband got home and things became more hectic. That became her flow, and I love when moms figure this out for themselves and feel confident in their decision.

Another mom started off pumping because her baby was born early and went to the NICU. Her goal was to get the baby off the bottle and back to the breast. She did all the therapies and homework we recommended, and approaching six weeks, her baby started nursing more frequently and gaining weight with just breastfeeding. She was thrilled—this was her journey, going from bottle to breast.

Then there was a third-time mom who had breastfed her first two babies successfully. With her third baby, she experienced persistent clogged ducts, engorgement, and oversupply, and her baby had reflux and gas issues. She decided, "You know what, I'm done. I don't want to nurse anymore. This is causing me way too much stress." She had three kids, needed to return to work soon, and made the decision that would give her the most peace. That was her finding her flow.

Recognizing Your Progress and Building Confidence

One challenge I see often is moms forgetting how far they've come. When I work with patients, we track their progress carefully.

Remember when you first had your baby and felt insecure about feeding—how much to feed, when to feed? Look at how responsive you are now to your baby's cues. Think back to those early days: maybe you were only able to breastfeed once or twice a day, and now you're up to five times. Maybe you could only latch with help, but now you can do it independently. Perhaps you started with making just 8 ounces of milk per day, and six weeks later you're producing 21 ounces—that's nearly triple!

Remember overcoming engorgement? How your breasts were so hard and tender? You did that. You can do hard things. If you had nipple pain, maybe it was a seven out of ten every single feed with damage. Now you might get an occasional pinch at a two or three out of ten, and your nipples look amazing. These are real victories.

Most moms tell me that getting regular support and validation is what helps them transition from those challenging early weeks to feeling more confident. It's incredibly important to have someone who can affirm what you're experiencing—someone who can say, "Yeah, I see what you're saying, you're 100 percent right, this is totally different behavior than last week." Having that confirmation that you're not imagining things and that you're actually learning your baby's patterns makes a huge difference.

> **Rule of Thumb:** Keep a simple feeding journal for a week or two when you're feeling uncertain about your progress. Looking back at where you started versus where you are now can provide a powerful perspective when you're having a tough day.

When parents come to me stressed about their baby's behavior or feeding patterns, I remind them of something important: your baby isn't going to be seventeen years old looking back and saying, "Mom, you didn't breastfeed me right, and so I'm messed up now." Our whole goal is to have a well-loved baby and provide proper nutrients however possible—not to put undue pressure on ourselves.

Finding Your Flow: Your Journey, Your Way

After thousands of hours supporting new mothers, I've learned that finding your flow means discovering what works best for you and your baby rather than reaching some magical perfect state. It's about learning new techniques each day, adapting to your baby's changing needs, and gradually building your confidence with each passing week.

Remember those early days when leaving the house seemed impossible? When every feeding felt like a mountain to climb? Look at you now. Whether you're exclusively breastfeeding, combining breast and bottle, or have found a completely different flow that works for your family, you've come so far.

As we wrap up this book, I'm going to say it again: your worth is not measured in ounces. It's measured in the love, dedication, and courage you show every day as you nurture your little one. This journey is yours. Not Instagram's, not your friend's, not your mother-in-law's—yours. Own it. Celebrate it. Trust it. And most importantly, trust yourself. You know your baby better than anyone else, and you're exactly the mother your baby needs.

Keep this book close, refer back to it when you need support, and remember: you've got this, mama!

ONE LAST MESSAGE

As we come to the close of our journey together, I want to thank you for letting me be a part of this chapter in your life. The first few weeks of breastfeeding that we've explored throughout this book are just the beginning of a beautiful, evolving relationship between you and your little one. What comes next is entirely yours to discover and shape, mama.

Remember that the support doesn't end when you close this book. I'd love to continue being part of your breastfeeding journey through The Boob Business Podcast, where we dive deeper into many of the topics we've touched on here. If you find yourself facing new challenges or simply want more personalized guidance, my team at Milk Diva is always here to help—whether through virtual consultations or in-person support if you're in or near Austin, Texas. And if you've found value in what you've learned, consider sharing your story with other moms who might be struggling. Your experience might be exactly what another mother needs to hear.

So as you move forward beyond these first crucial weeks, keep nurturing, keep loving, and keep believing in yourself. You are doing an incredible job, mama, and I'm cheering you on every step of the way.

With all my love and support,
Naiomi S. Catron

INSIDER
RESOURCES
FINDING YOUR FLOW IN THE FIRST WEEKS OF BREASTFEEDING
MILK'D
NAIOMI CATRON
SCAN
ME!

ACKNOWLEDGMENTS

To God,

I am forever grateful for the divine guidance and inspiration You have given to me. Thank You for igniting within me the deep-seated passion to care for women during their most delicate and precious moments of motherhood. Your unwavering presence and grace have been my guiding light.

To My Amazing Husband, Christian,

Your unwavering love, boundless encouragement, and attentive ear have been my steadfast pillars of support. Thank you for standing by my side, for sharing in my journey, and for being my rock through every twist and turn.

To My Awesome Sons, Elijah & Caleb,

As you guys grow into amazing young men, I can't help but feel incredibly proud and thankful. Being your mom has been the absolute best, shaping me in ways I never expected. Thanks for showing me what true love, grit, and determination really mean. You both bring so much joy and laughter into my world, and I'm beyond grateful for the privilege of being your mom. Here's to your journeys ahead—may they be filled with endless opportunities, and always remember, my love for you knows no limits.

To My Favorite Mother-in-Law, Zenaida,

Your unwavering belief in my dreams and your unwavering encouragement have lifted me up in moments of doubt and uncertainty. Your faith in me has been a source of strength and inspiration.

To My Cherished Parents, Lillian & Nelson,

Your endless sacrifices and tireless dedication have paved the way for my dreams to flourish. Thank you for your unwavering love, for providing me with a nurturing environment to grow and thrive, and for instilling in me the values of perseverance and resilience. You are the true heroes of my story, and I am forever grateful for your boundless love and support.

To My Beloved Grandmother, Angelina,

Abuela, you were the rock of our family, and your legacy lives on in all of us. Your prayers were like a shield of protection, guiding me through life's ups and downs and helping me reach my fullest potential. Your unwavering faith and love continue to inspire me every day. Thank you for being my guardian angel and for blessing my life with your endless love and prayers. Te amo para siempre.

Through the years, many people have shared ideas, mentoring, and support that have impacted my life, each in a different way. It's impossible to thank everyone, and I apologize to anyone not listed. Please know that I appreciate you greatly. I want to extend my deepest gratitude to those who have mentored and guided me with unwavering dedication, helping me to become the professional I am today.

To Autumn R. Henning, MS, CCC-SLP, COM, IBCLC,

Thank you for your innovative approach to collaborative care and for being a trailblazer in the field of tongue-tie management. Your mentorship has been instrumental in helping me understand the complexities of oral function and how to best support families through their feeding challenges.

To Lisa Lahey, FNP-C, IBCLC, CSOM,

Your tireless work and commitment to the lactation field and your family have been a source of inspiration for me. Your passion for helping families, coupled with your extensive knowledge, has guided me in providing the best care possible to my own patients.

To Dr. Katrina Mitchell, MD, IBCLC, PMH-C

Thank you for your compassionate approach to patient care and your invaluable contributions to the field of breastfeeding medicine. Your work has helped shape my understanding of how to support mothers not just physically, but emotionally, through the postpartum period.

To Dr. Jared Poplin, DMD

Your expertise and dedication in the field of pediatric dentistry and optimizing oral health, have greatly influenced my approach to treating babies with tongue ties. Thank you for your collaborative spirit and for always putting the needs of the smallest patients first.

To all the incredible people who have worked at Milk Diva,

I have learned so much from each of you. Your dedication, hard work, and passion for helping families have not only shaped our practice but have also taught me invaluable lessons along the way. Thank you for being part of this journey and for contributing to the success of our team.

To anyone who has ever taken the time to teach, mentor, or simply offer a word of encouragement,

Thank you. Your tireless and often thankless work has made an indelible impact on my life and the lives of countless families. This book is a testament to the knowledge and wisdom you've imparted to me.

Finally, to all the mothers and babies who have allowed me to be a part of their journey,

You are the reason I do what I do. Thank you for trusting me to guide you through some of the most precious and challenging moments of your lives. This book is for you!

READY FOR PERSONALIZED LACTATION SUPPORT?

Whether you're local to Austin or joining us from afar, we're here to support your breastfeeding journey every step of the way.

If you're in the Austin area, you can book your in-person appointment with our expert team by visiting www.milkdiva.com or scan this QR code:

Not local? No worries!

We offer virtual prenatal courses and one-on-one virtual consultations to help you prepare for a smooth feeding journey, no matter where you are.

Explore our offerings at www.milkdiva.com/lactation-services to get started or scan this QR code:

Let's work together to ensure you and your baby have the best start possible!

P.S. Please understand, we usually have at least a 1–2-week waitlist so contact us while you are still pregnant!

THE IDEAL SPEAKER FOR YOUR NEXT EVENT

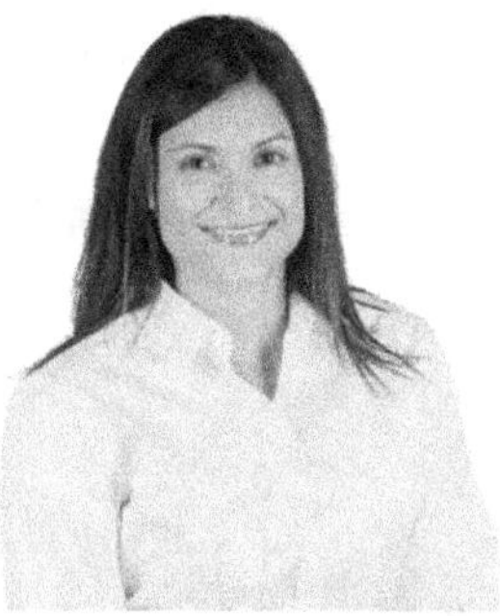

Are you looking for a speaker who blends clinical expertise, real-life experience, and a passion for supporting both families and wellness professionals? I'd be honored to speak at your next event! Whether it's an educational workshop, a professional conference, or a business-focused seminar, I'd love to inspire your audience with actionable insights on:

- Building and Growing a Thriving Health & Wellness Practice
- Prenatal Education & Birth Preparedness
- Navigating Tongue Tie & Collaborative Care
- Breastfeeding Success & Overcoming Challenges
- Empowering Patient-Centered Care in Maternal Health

Let's collaborate to create a meaningful and impactful experience for your attendees. Reach out here: Info@milkdiva.com

ABOUT THE AUTHOR

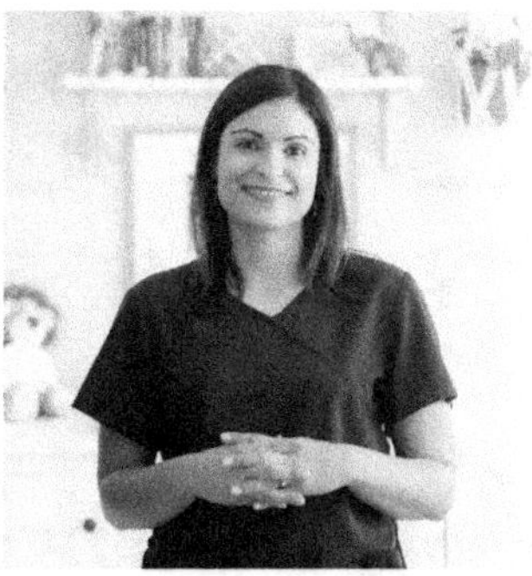

Naiomi S. Catron is a distinguished figure in lactation and infant feeding collaborative care. With a background as both an award-winning labor & delivery nurse and an International Board-Certified Lactation Consultant (IBCLC), Naiomi founded Milk Diva Lactation Services in Austin, TX in 2019. Her visionary leadership has not only established Milk Diva as a premier destination for lactation support but also transformed it into a thriving multi-provider and multi-disciplinary practice. Through her innovative approach, Naiomi has fostered a collaborative environment that significantly improves outcomes for breastfeeding families. Her dedication to identifying root causes and supporting families has earned her recognition as a trusted advocate for families facing breastfeeding issues including but not limited to tethered oral tissues (aka "tongue-ties"). Committed to her mission, Naiomi works tirelessly to foster thriving lactation practices and elevate the lactation profession, advocating for equal respect as allied healthcare professionals. Naiomi is a wife to Christian of 23 years (and counting) and mother of two college bound young men.

www.ingramcontent.com/pod-product-compliance
Lightning Source LLC
LaVergne TN
LVHW022214200926
848481LV00006B/1964